A Trip To THE STORE

How to choose and enjoy nutritious foods

By Florentina Marcu

"If it came from a plant, eat it; if it was made in a plant, don't." ~ Michael Pollan

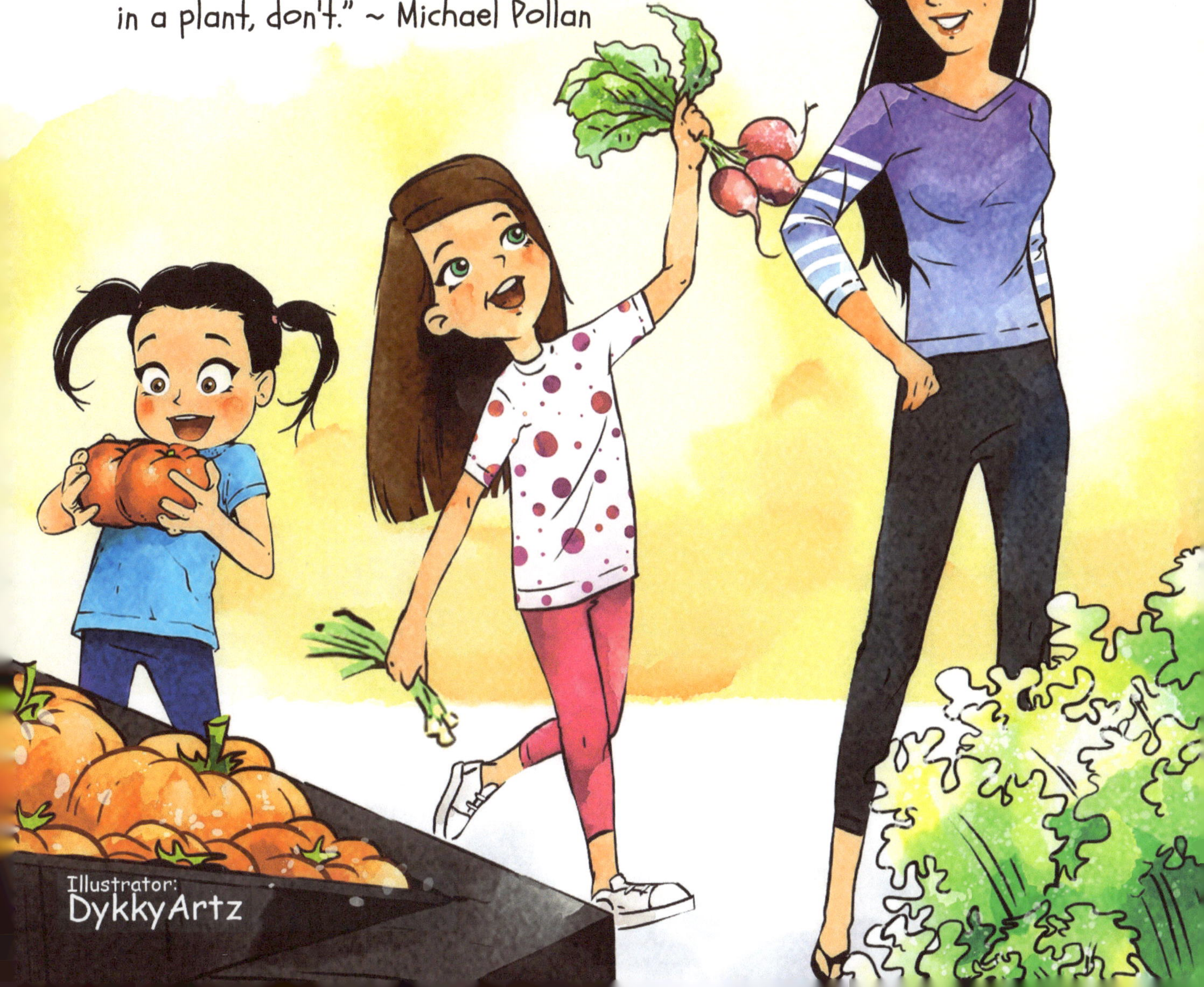

Illustrator: DykkyArtz

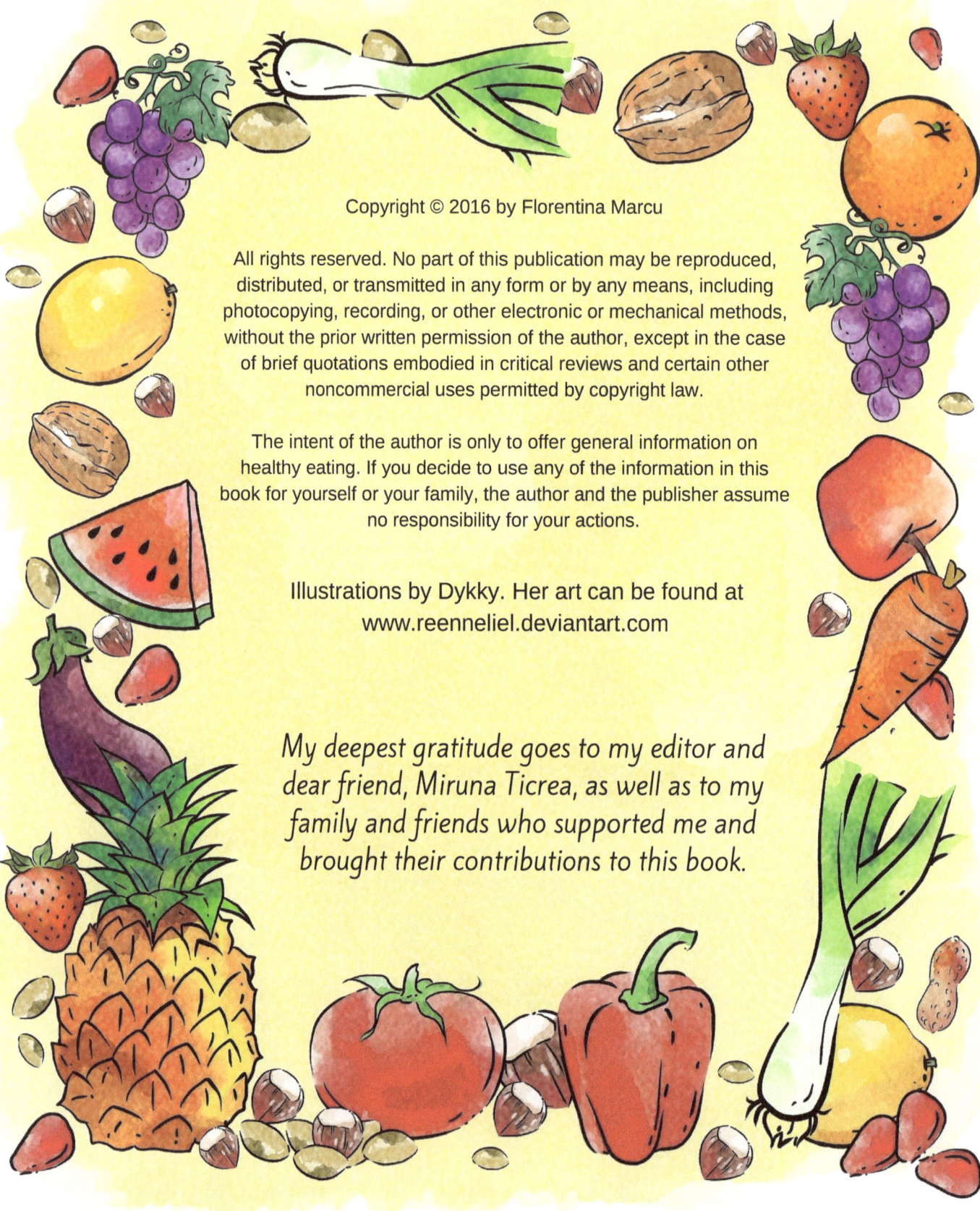

Copyright © 2016 by Florentina Marcu

All rights reserved. No part of this publication may be reproduced, distributed, or transmitted in any form or by any means, including photocopying, recording, or other electronic or mechanical methods, without the prior written permission of the author, except in the case of brief quotations embodied in critical reviews and certain other noncommercial uses permitted by copyright law.

The intent of the author is only to offer general information on healthy eating. If you decide to use any of the information in this book for yourself or your family, the author and the publisher assume no responsibility for your actions.

Illustrations by Dykky. Her art can be found at www.reenneliel.deviantart.com

My deepest gratitude goes to my editor and dear friend, Miruna Ticrea, as well as to my family and friends who supported me and brought their contributions to this book.

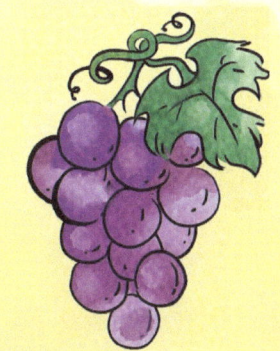

Dear Parents and Teachers,

As a health coach and mom, I always look for ways to feed my family nutritious foods to keep us healthy and strong. I wrote this book to teach kids the importance of always choosing real foods over highly processed foods. In today's world, it is quite a challenge to stay away from the multitude of processed food-like items, which offer convenience and come in colorful and attractive packages, but which are not the best choices for good health.

I would like to encourage you to read this book together with your child and discuss the topics as you go along. The earlier in life children learn about the importance of good nutrition, the more likely it is that they will embrace it for the rest of their lives. If they get into the habit of always checking the labels and deciphering the ingredients that make up the food they want to get, they will always choose the right foods for their health.

I remember one of my daughters calling me from the other side of an aisle in the store: "Mom, we shouldn't buy this because it has partially hydrogenated oil!" Of course I would get glances from people hearing this from a 6-year old, but the reality is that I only mentioned these undesirable ingredients to them once or twice, and they got it. Kids learn very quickly and if you take the time to explain things, they will understand that some foods are better for them than others.

When children gain the knowledge in this book and are involved in the process of choosing their foods and preparing their meals, you will discover that they like certain healthful foods that you didn't even think about serving to them. My younger daughter snatched a bunch of rainbow chard when we were at the store one time, and she ate it like that once we washed it at home. It looked so colorful and fresh to her that she didn't think it needed any preparation! My older daughter now has celery root on her snack list. That is because she was helping me to chop veggies for a soup one day and she wanted to taste the chopped raw celery root. She loved it and now we serve it often (as is or with a little homemade mayonnaise)!

It is my hope that this book will help you start a dialogue in your family and inspire you to make better choices when it comes to food. Foods that grow in nature are real foods and are best for your body. Mother Nature knows best!

In good health,

Florentina

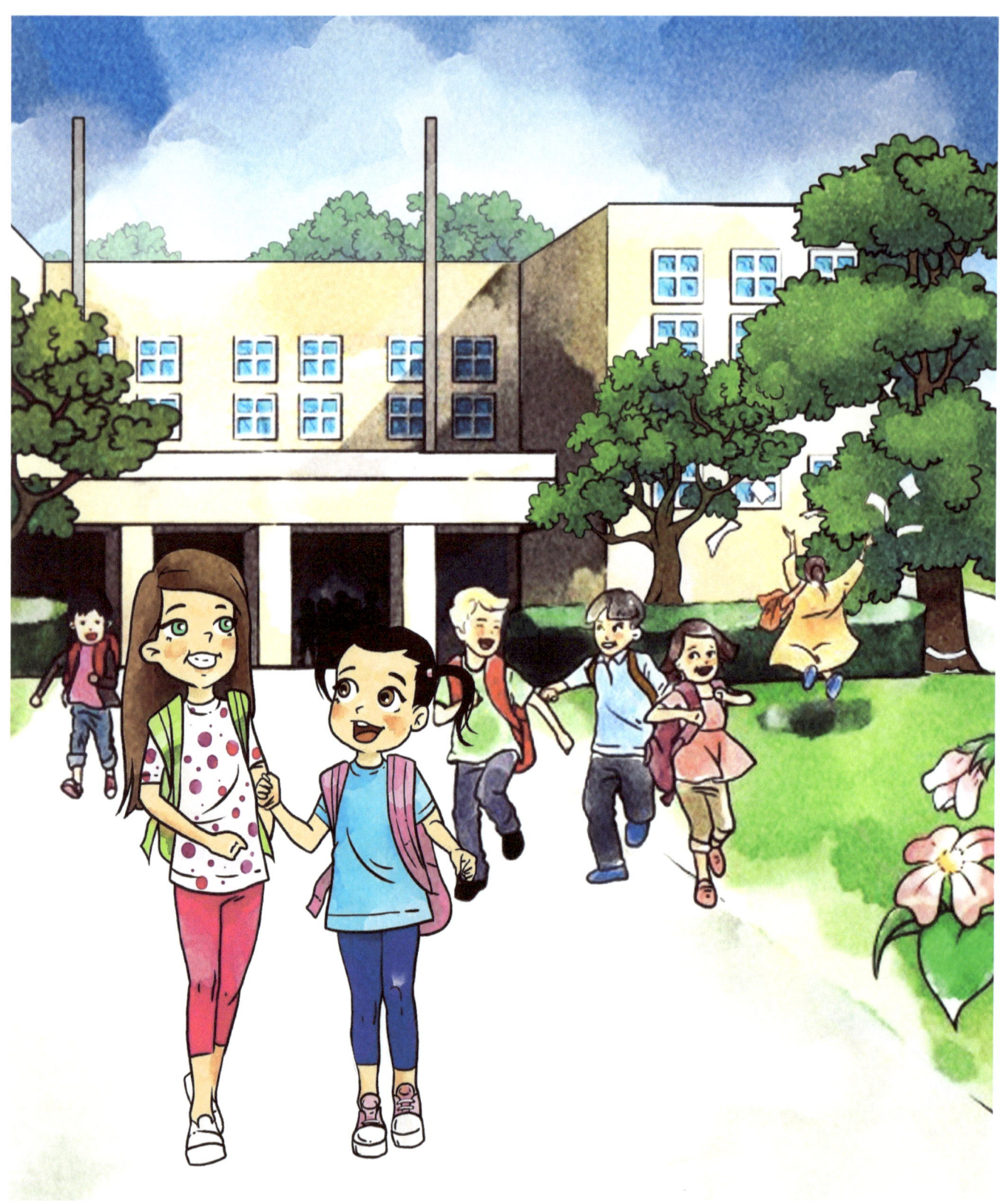

"Yay, school is over!" It was Friday afternoon and the kids were ready for the weekend.

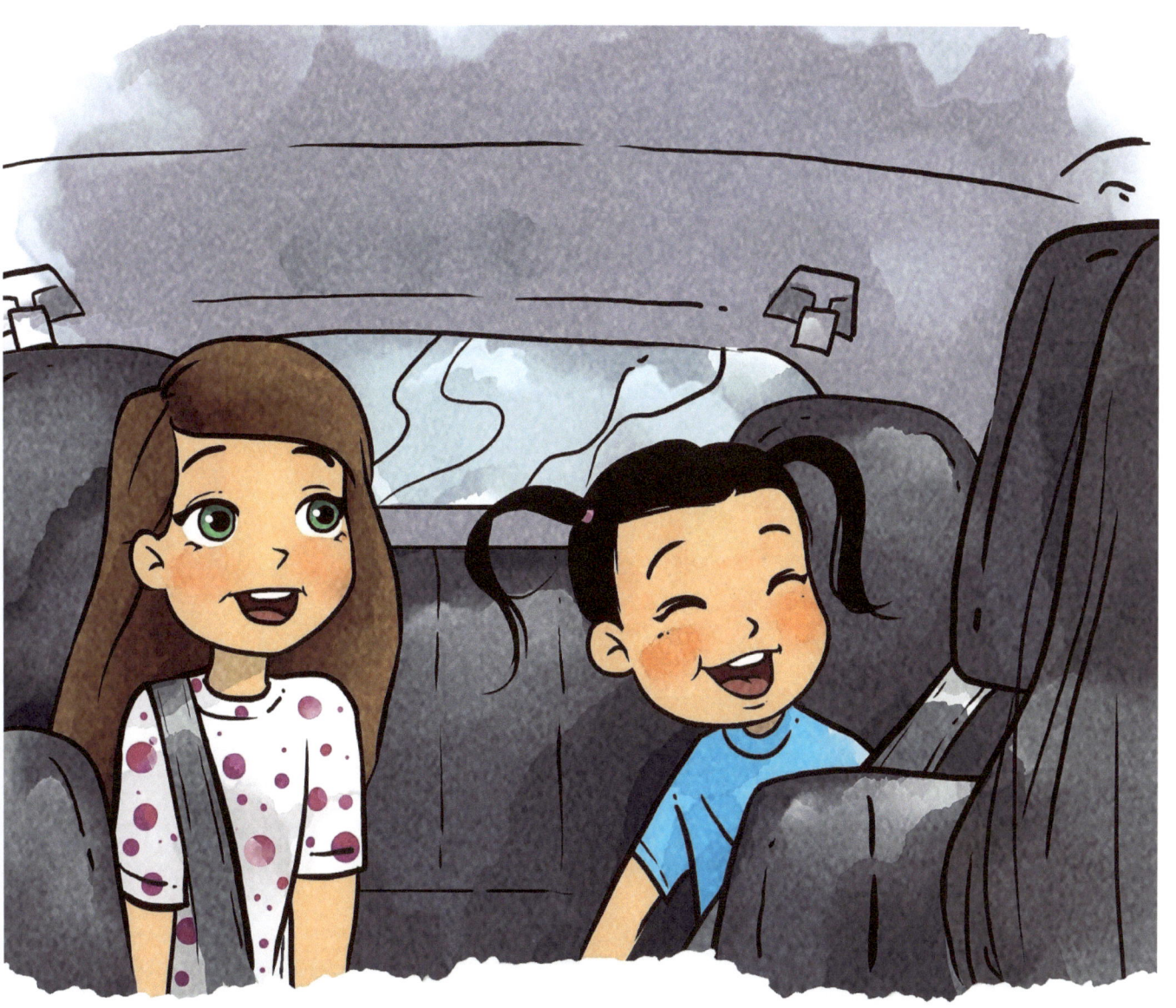

Maya and Zara got into their Mom's car and said, almost with one voice, "Can we go to the store and buy some yummy food?"

"Actually," Mom said, "I was going to ask you the same thing! I have a list of things we need to buy for the weekend."

"Oh, I'm sure we'll add to the list, Mom..." Maya said.

At the store, they went over to the fresh produce section. "What do we need to get?" asked Zara.

"Well, let's start with a salad," Mom said, as she picked a big, fresh head of red butter lettuce. "What would you like to add to the salad?" she asked.

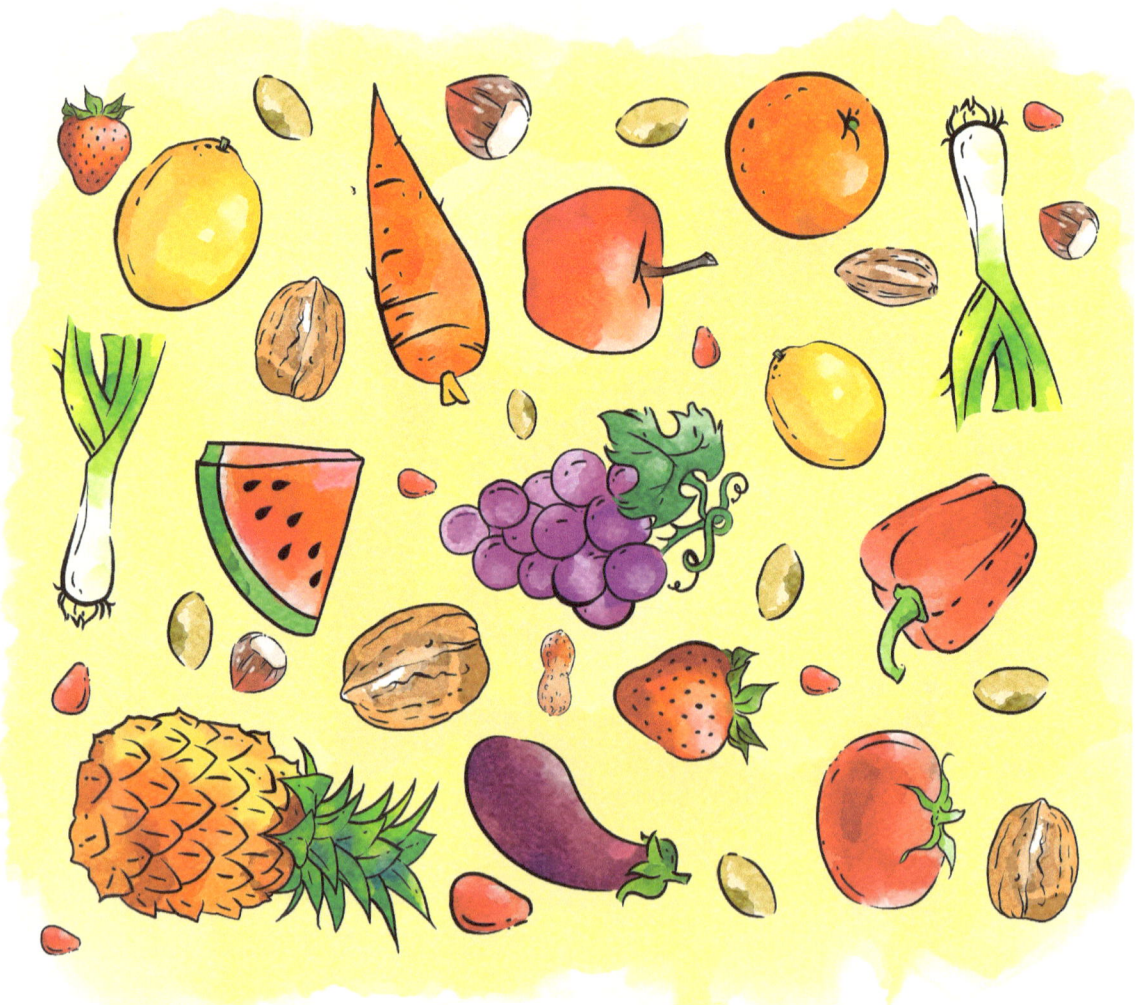

Maya picked a bunch of green onions, another one of radishes, and some red peppers.

Zara picked a head of cauliflower, cucumbers, and some heirloom tomatoes. "These are my favorite!" she said, holding two shiny, plump tomatoes.

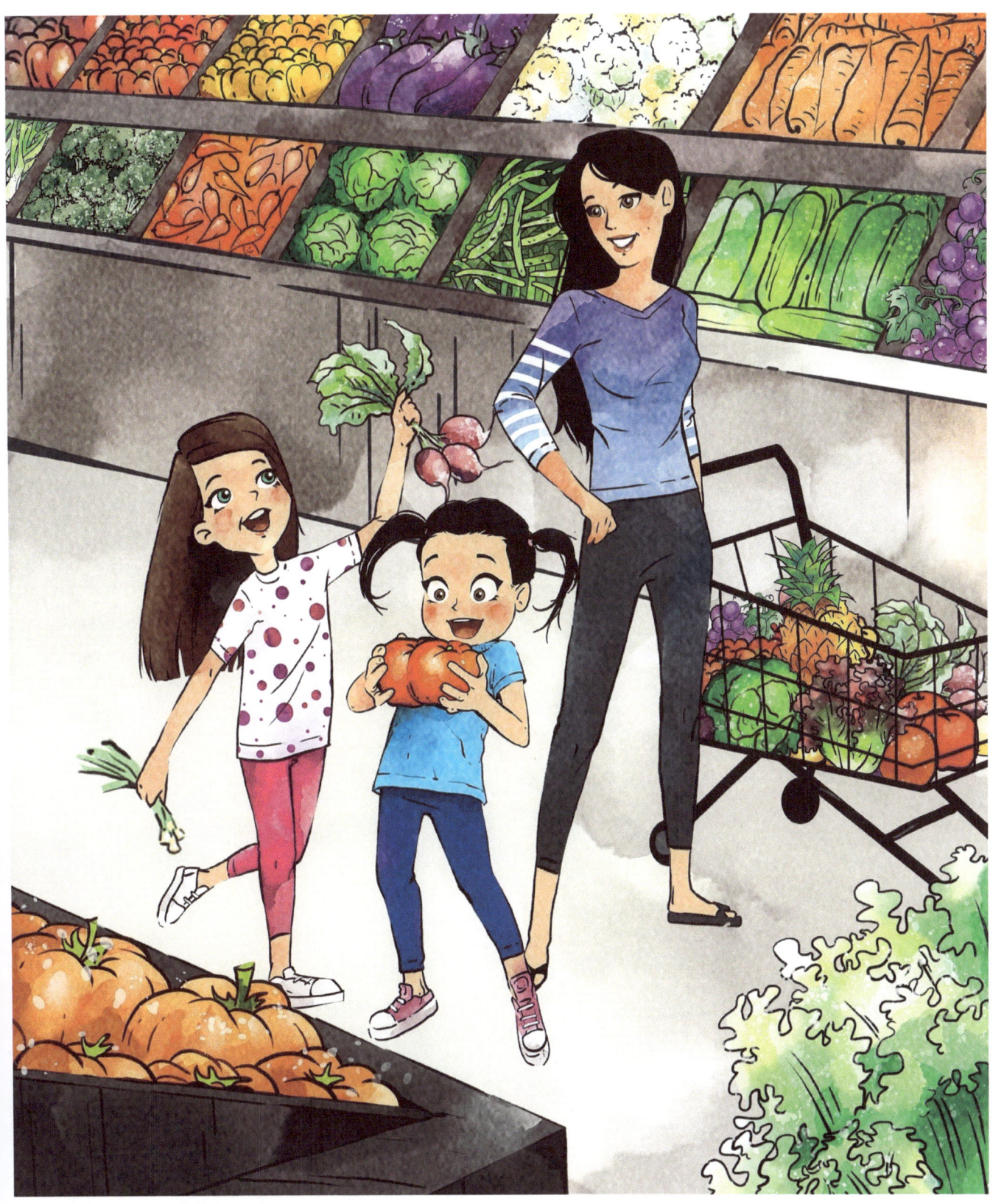

All of the vegetables looked so fresh and colorful!

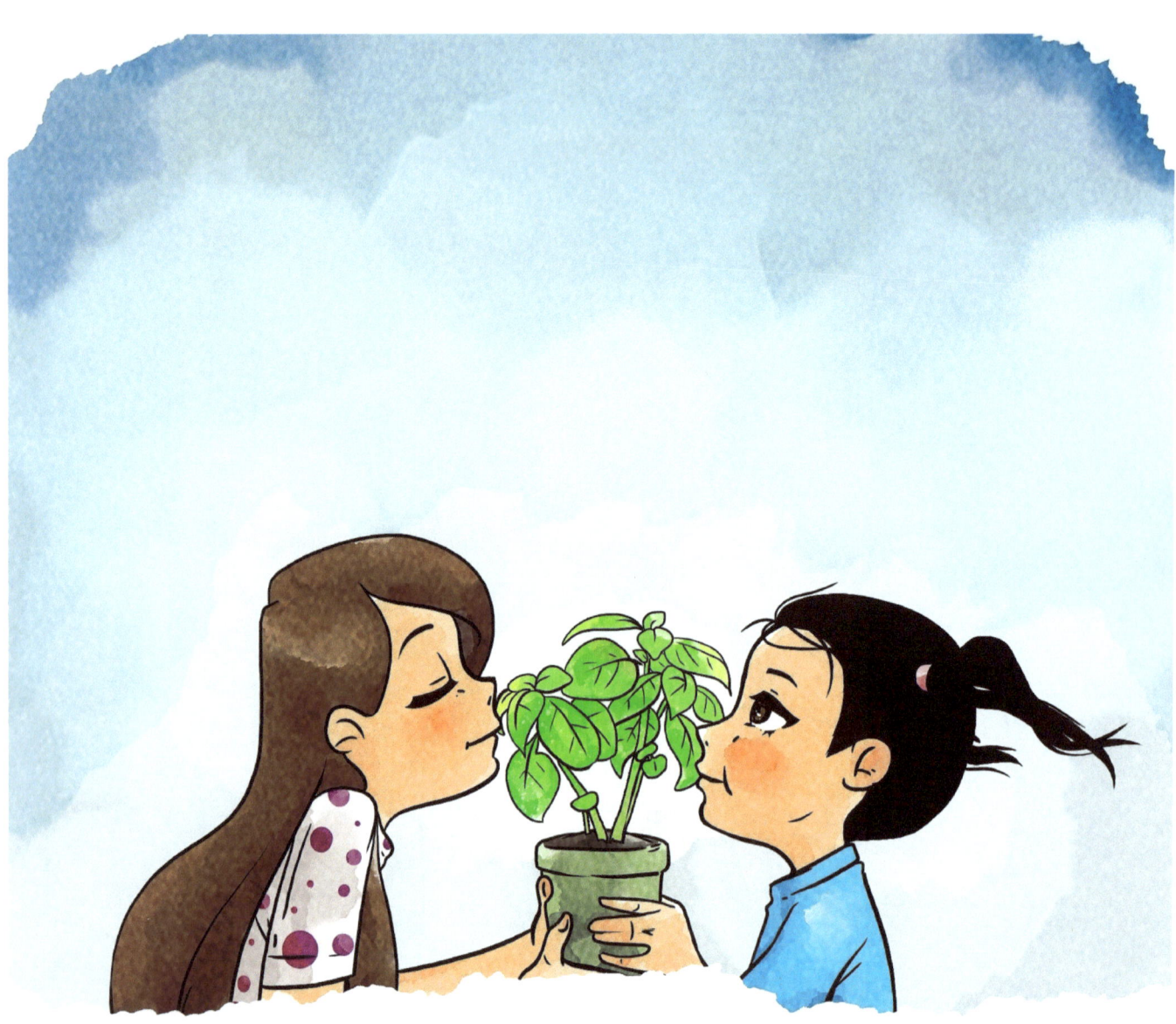

"OK, all our salad needs now is some fresh parsley," Mom said. "And let's get some fresh basil as well, to make a nice dressing."

The girls wanted to sniff the basil, as they always do. They just loved the sweet aroma of this herb.

"Can we bake fish for dinner tonight?" suggested Maya.

"That's a good idea and it's quick to make," said Mom. "We can get some wild salmon and put it in the oven with a bit of butter and minced garlic. Then we serve it with lemon juice and the salad."

"And mashed potatoes!" added Zara.

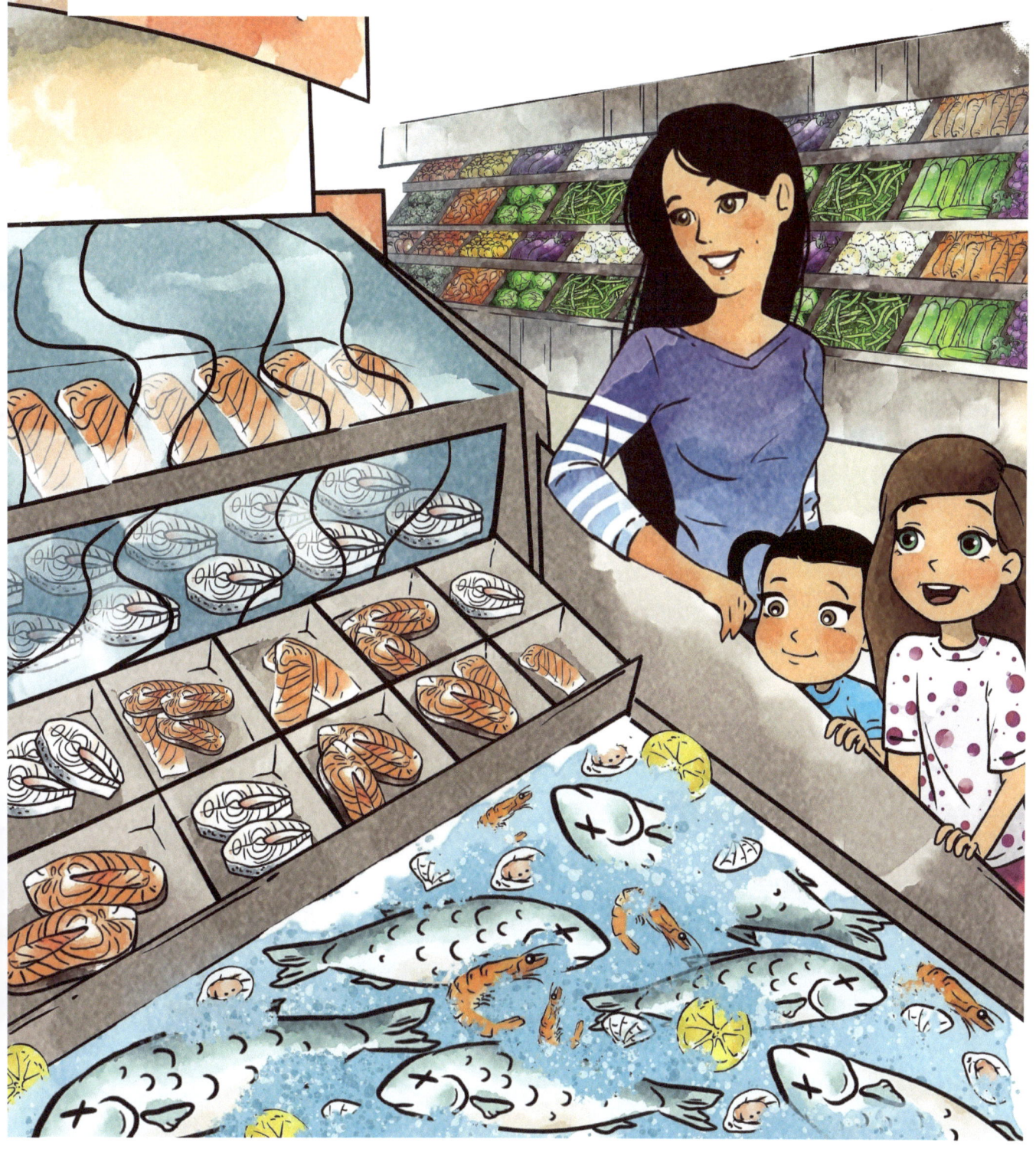

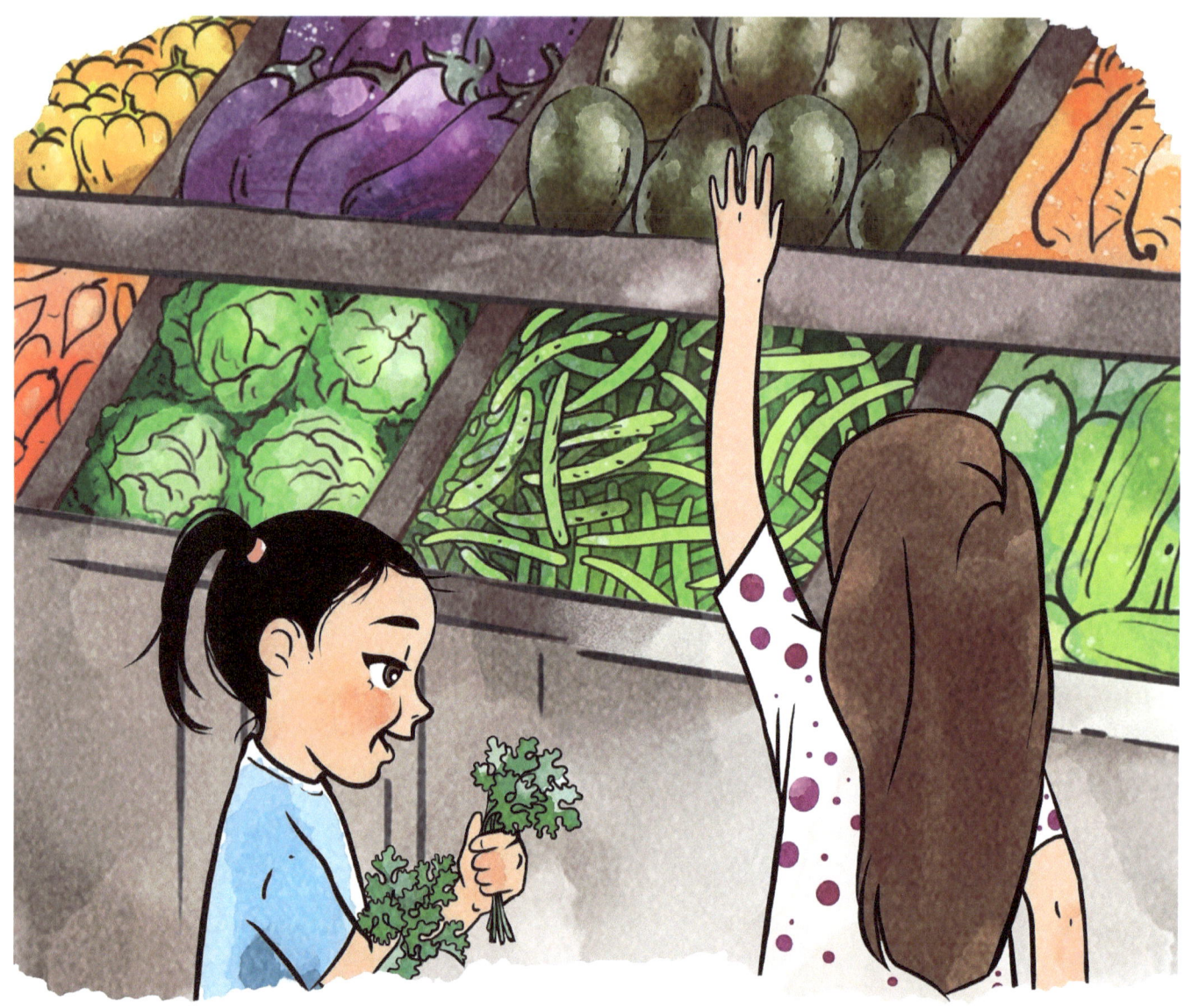

"What would you like to have for dinner tomorrow?" Mom asked. "Should we make tacos?"

"Yes! They are our favorite!" the girls said.

"Then let's get some ground turkey and tortillas. We also need avocados and red onions to make guacamole, as well as fresh cilantro, garlic, and limes to make salsa."

The girls were going in different directions picking all of the items.

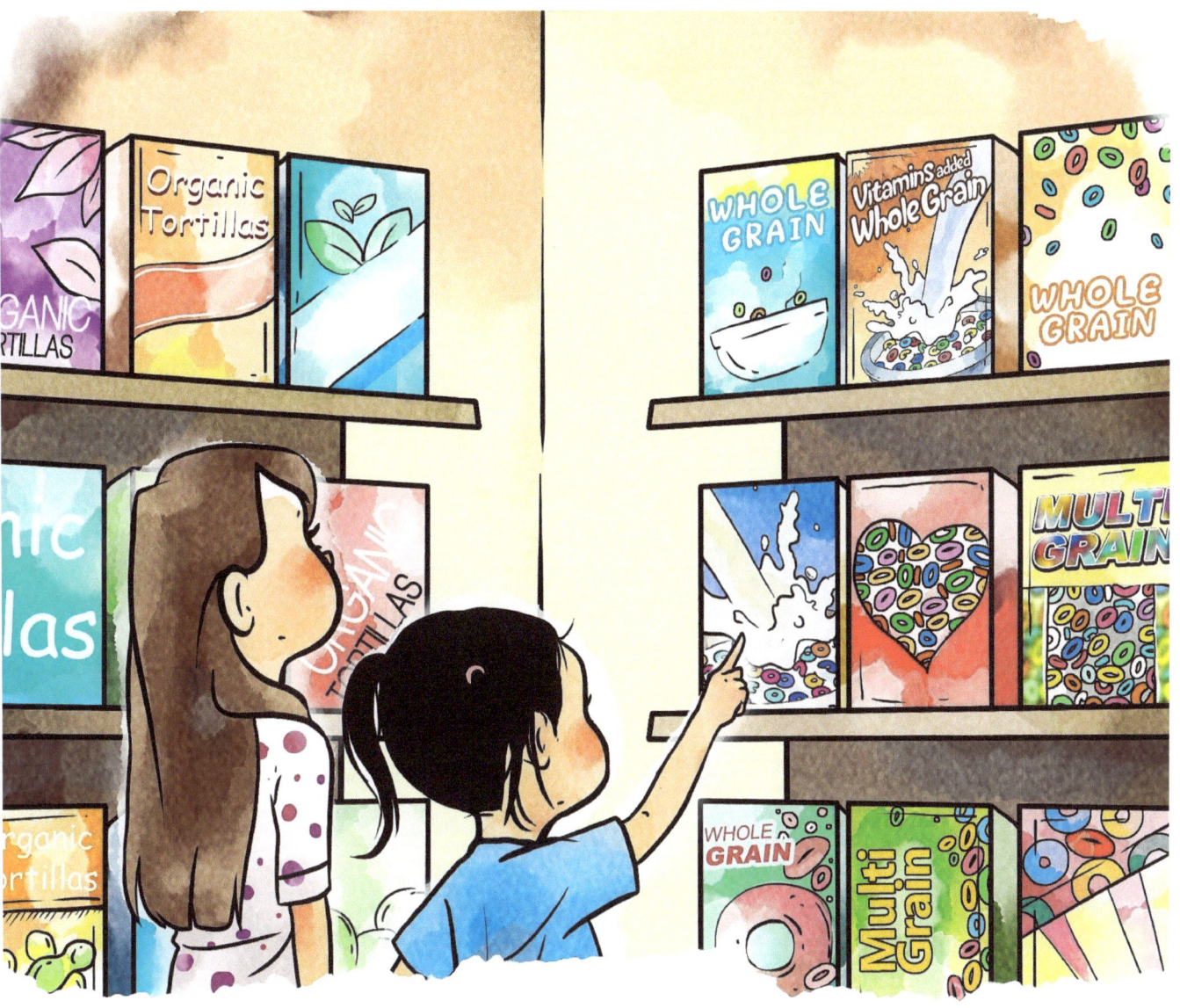

As they were looking for their favorite spelt tortillas, Zara spotted a colorful box of breakfast cereal. "Should we get this?" she asked.

"What do we do when we want to buy packaged foods?" Mom asked, smiling.

"We check the ingredients!" the girls answered.

"In general, we try to buy most of our food from the perimeter of the store. This is where all of the fresh produce is found and this is what we call real foods."

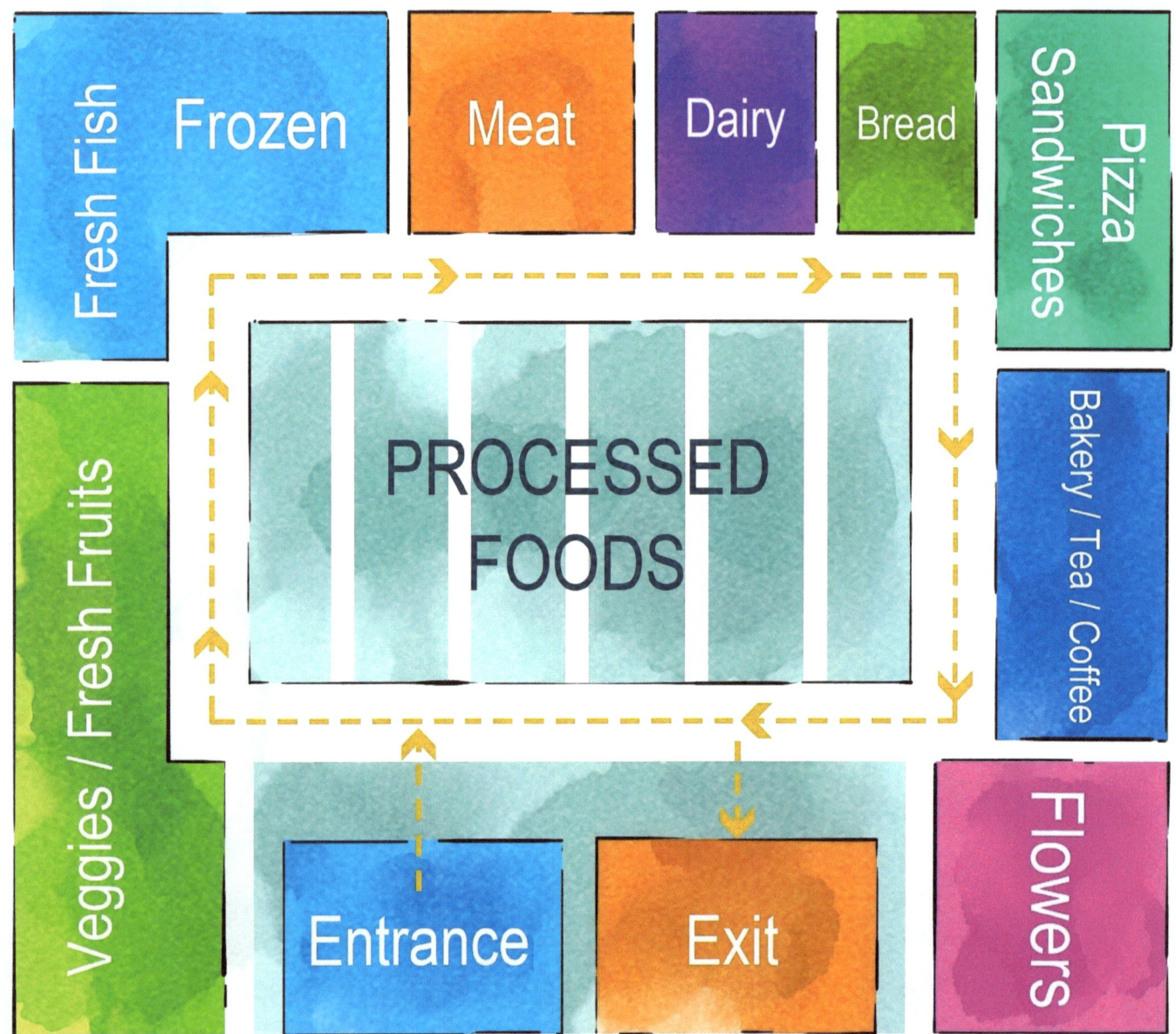

"Can you give me some examples of real foods?" Mom asked.

"Kale, bananas, and eggs!" Maya said.

"Carrots, pumpkin seeds, and fish!" Zara added.

"Yes! Foods that grow in nature are real foods and they are nourishing to our bodies!" Mom agreed.

"Now, you may ask, aren't all of the foods in a grocery store real foods? You can find a lot of *food-like* items that we call processed foods and that we want to avoid. They come in all kinds of packaging, like this cereal box, and are manufactured in a facility."

"Most often, processed foods have nutrients taken out. For example, many breads are made with refined flour and have little to no fiber, to make those breads softer and last more on the shelves."

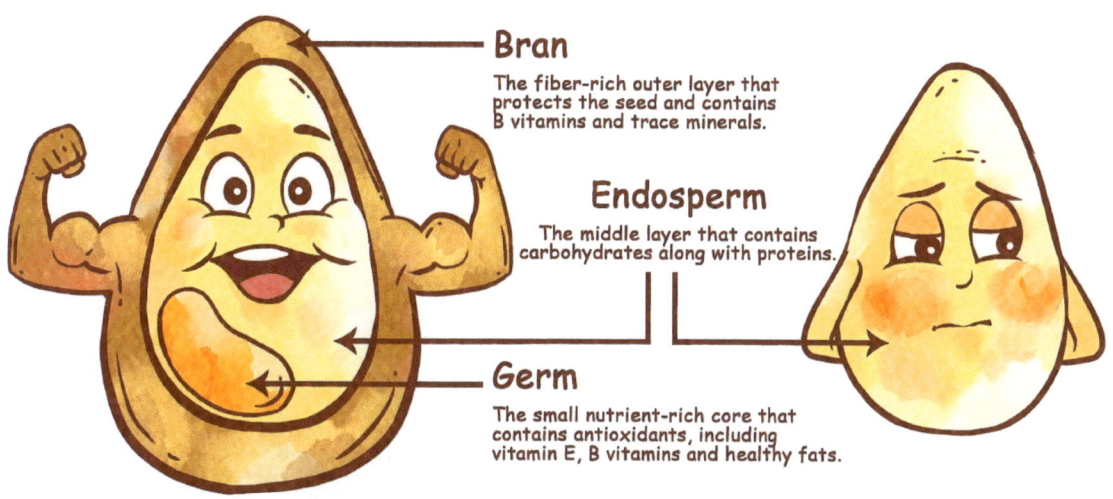

Whole Grain vs. Refined Grain

Bran
The fiber-rich outer layer that protects the seed and contains B vitamins and trace minerals.

Endosperm
The middle layer that contains carbohydrates along with proteins.

Germ
The small nutrient-rich core that contains antioxidants, including vitamin E, B vitamins and healthy fats.

"Natural whole grains contain fiber and many nutrients that are important for good health. When we buy foods made of grains, we want to get at least 2 grams of fiber per serving. So we check the label to make sure that sugar is low, but fiber is high," Mom explained.

"What about all of those vitamins and minerals that are added to certain foods, such as breads and cereals?" Maya asked. "Don't they make the food better?"

"The reason those vitamins and minerals are added to the foods is because those foods were stripped of their nutrition in the first place," Mom said. "We want wholesome foods that don't need any vitamins or minerals added, since they already contain those in their natural version."

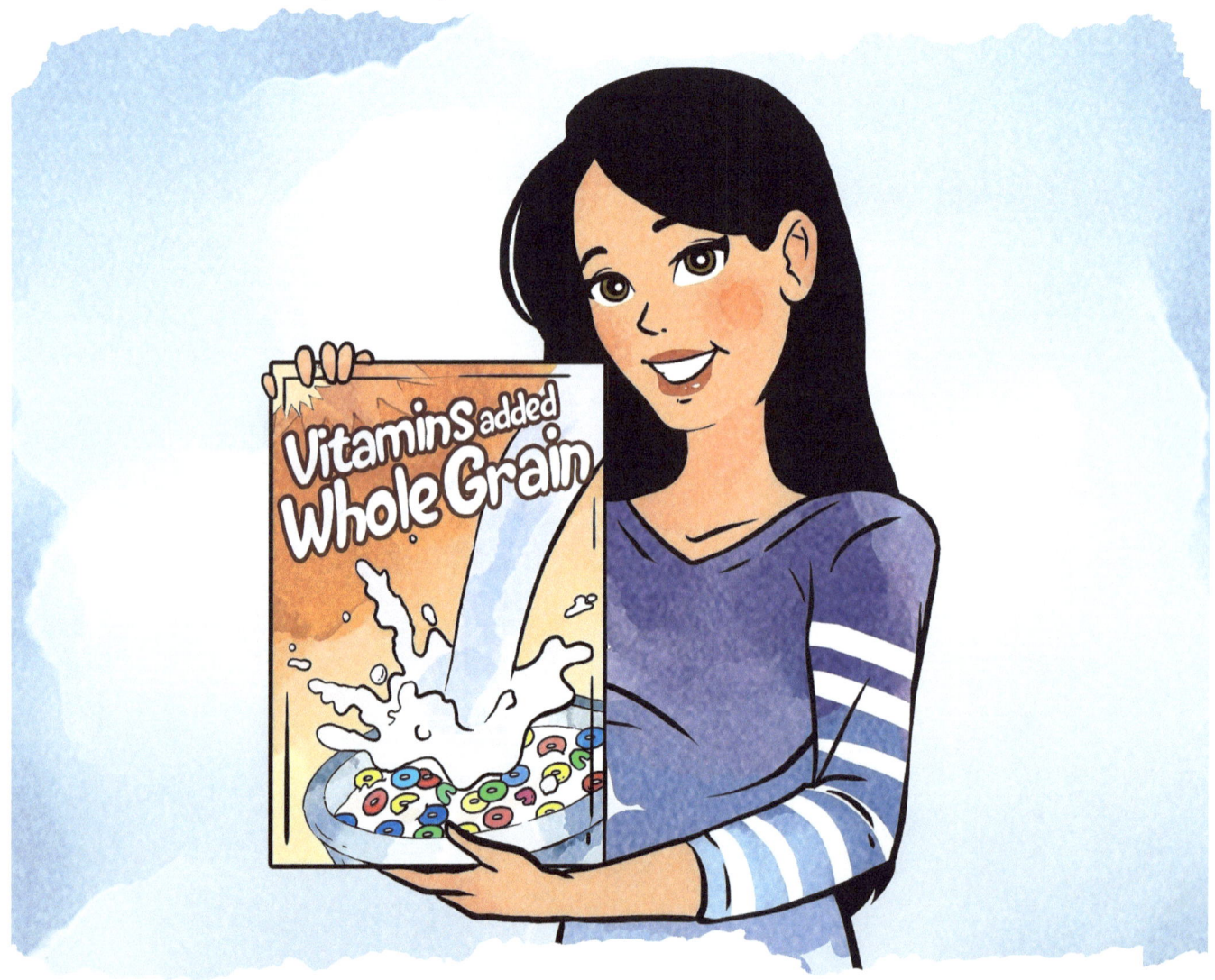

"Mother Nature knows best, and our bodies assimilate better nutrients that are naturally found in foods. When we see foods made with refined, bromated, or even enriched flour, for example, we know those foods were highly processed and are not the best choices for us."

"Now, let's check the ingredient list on this cereal box. On the front it says that the cereal contains whole grains and has added vitamins. But we know that the Nutrition Facts label and the Ingredient list on the back or the side of the box are the things we need to check," said Mom. "What are we looking for when we check the ingredient list?"

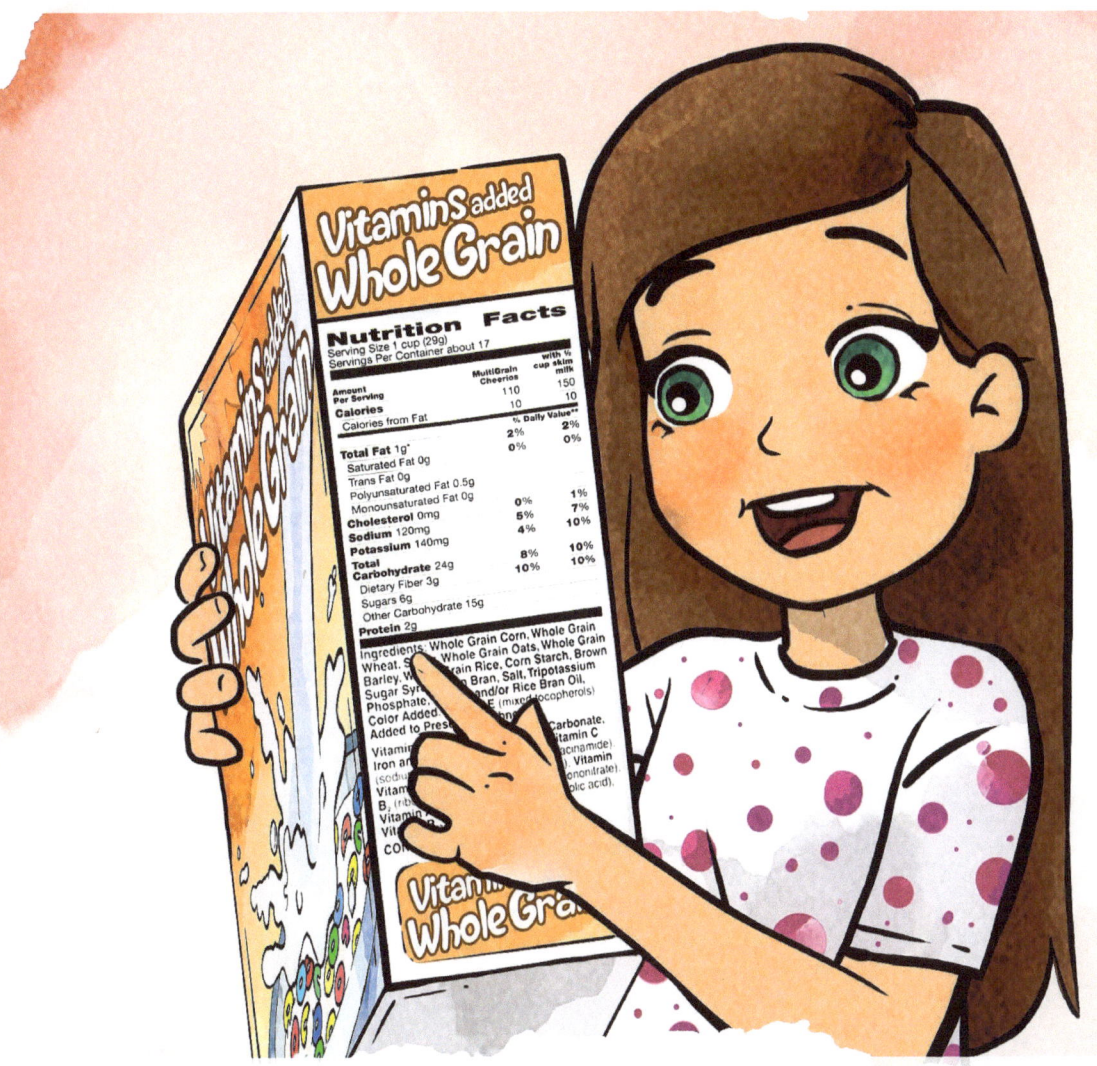

"The first ingredient on the list is the most important because that's what's mostly in the food," Maya said.

"That's right!" Mom said, "Ingredients are listed in the order of their quantity. The more of an ingredient is in the food, the closer to the top of the list it is. So we wouldn't buy cereal that has sugar or refined flour as the first ingredients, even if it says *Whole Grain* on the front of the box."

"But I like sweet foods!" Zara said smiling.

"Of course you do. I do, too! But we have to avoid too much added sugar to keep our bodies healthy and strong!" Mom said.

"And our teeth will be healthy and strong, too, if we don't eat too much sugar and processed foods," Maya added.

"We can always enjoy fruits and sweet vegetables such as pumpkin or carrots, or we can make our own desserts using wholesome ingredients and less sugar," added Mom.

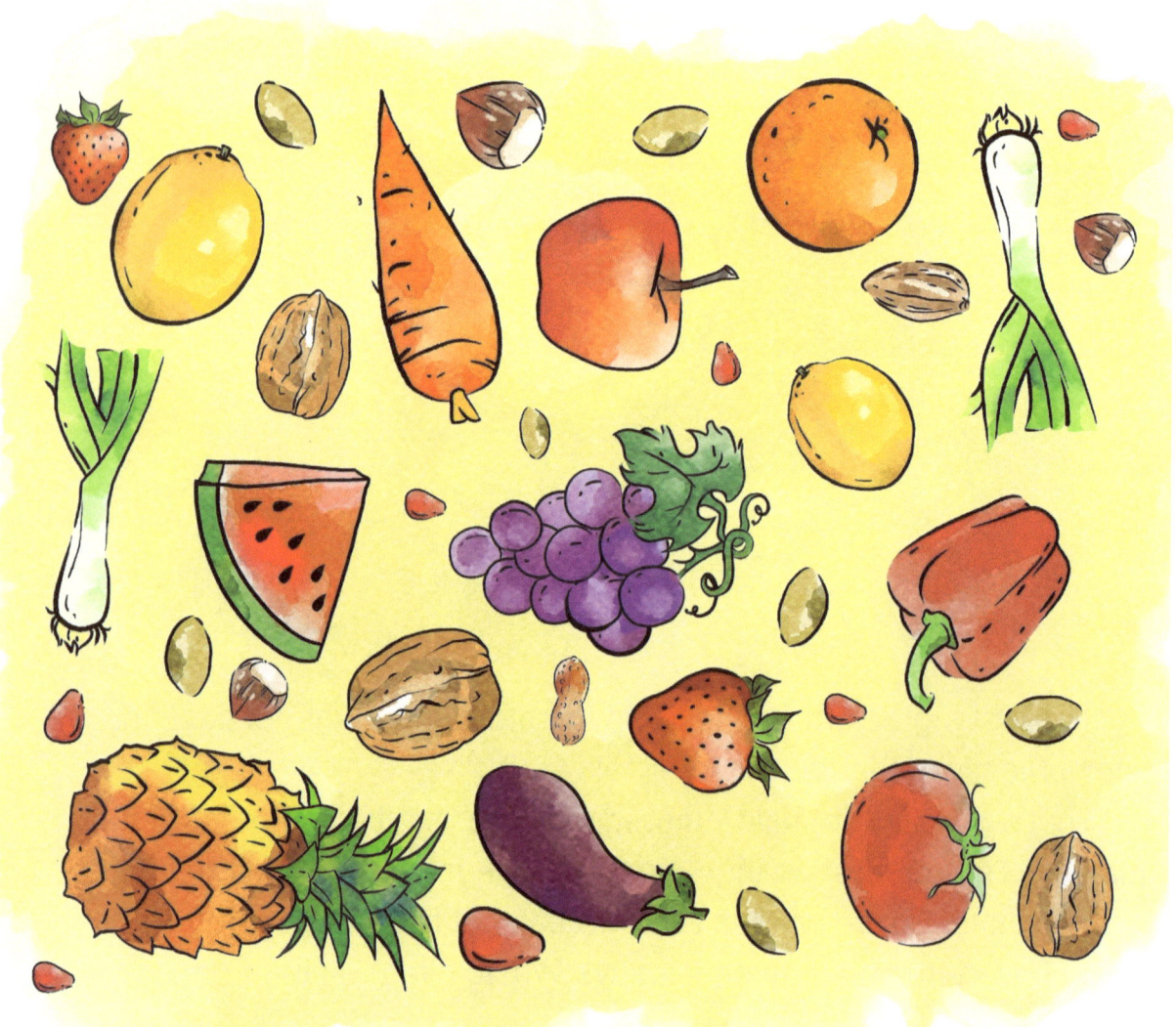

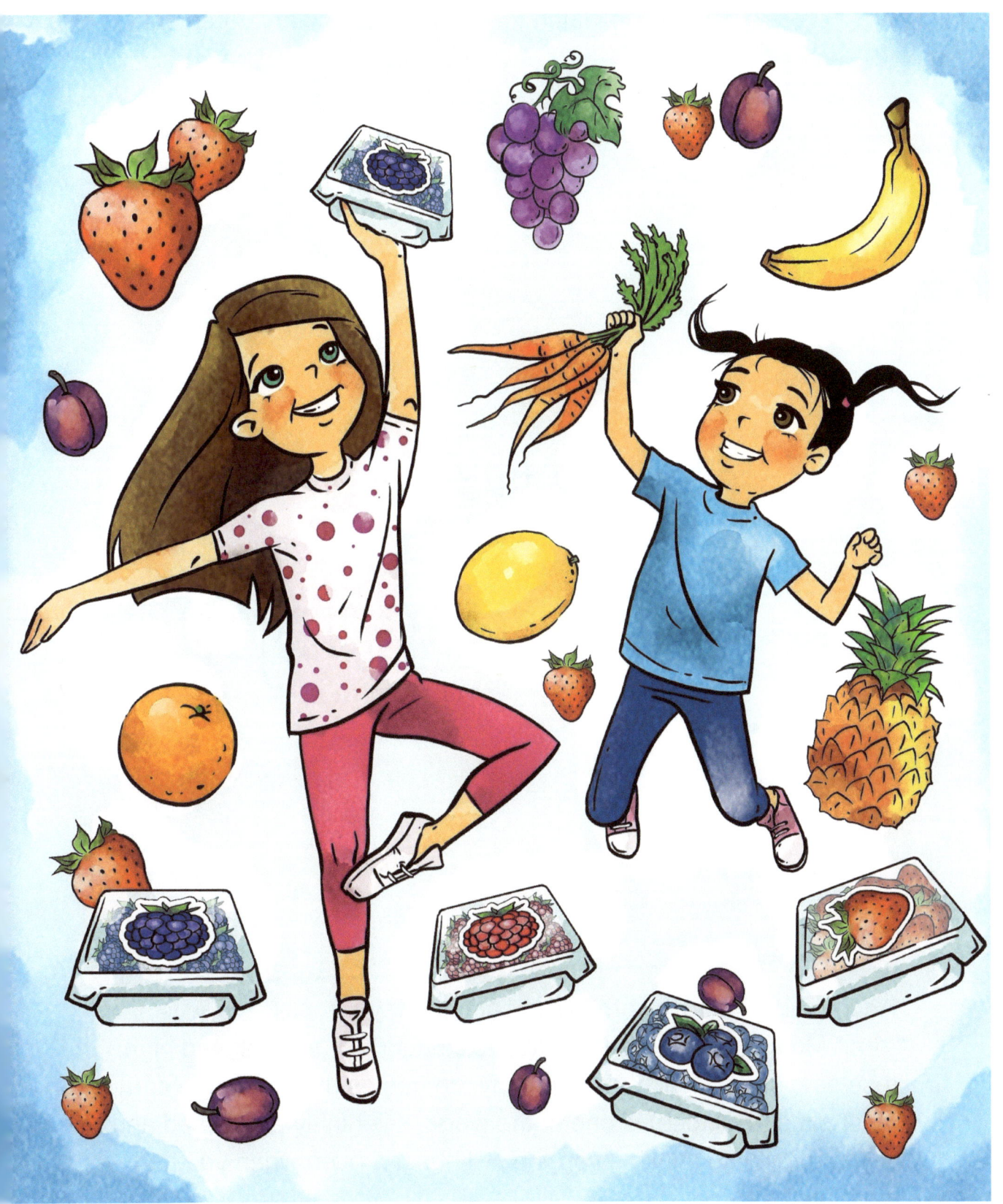

"What else do we have to watch for when we check an ingredient list?" asked Mom.

"Partially hydrogenated oils!" Zara said.

"Yes," Mom said, "Those are also called trans fats, and they are not good for the heart."

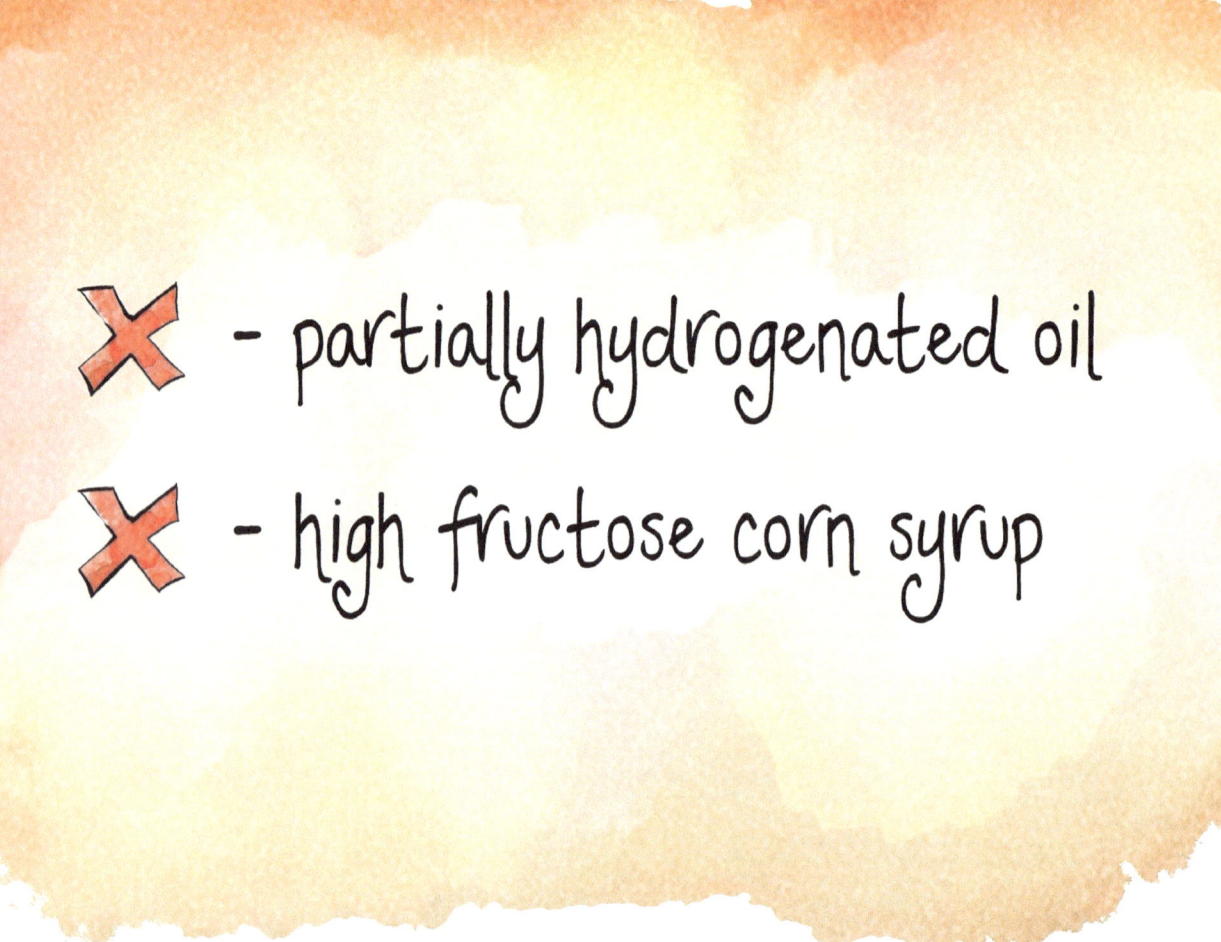

X - partially hydrogenated oil

X - high fructose corn syrup

"And no high fructose corn syrup," added Maya.

"Yes," Mom agreed, "We have to avoid sugars in general, and high fructose corn syrup (which also goes by the names of corn sugar, corn syrup, or simply fructose) is one of the worst. It is highly processed and it tricks your brain into thinking you are still hungry, even when you had plenty to eat!"

"One way to limit your sugar is to avoid sugary drinks, such as sodas and fruit juices. Most of them contain a lot of sugar and other questionable ingredients. What is the best beverage you can drink?" asked Mom.

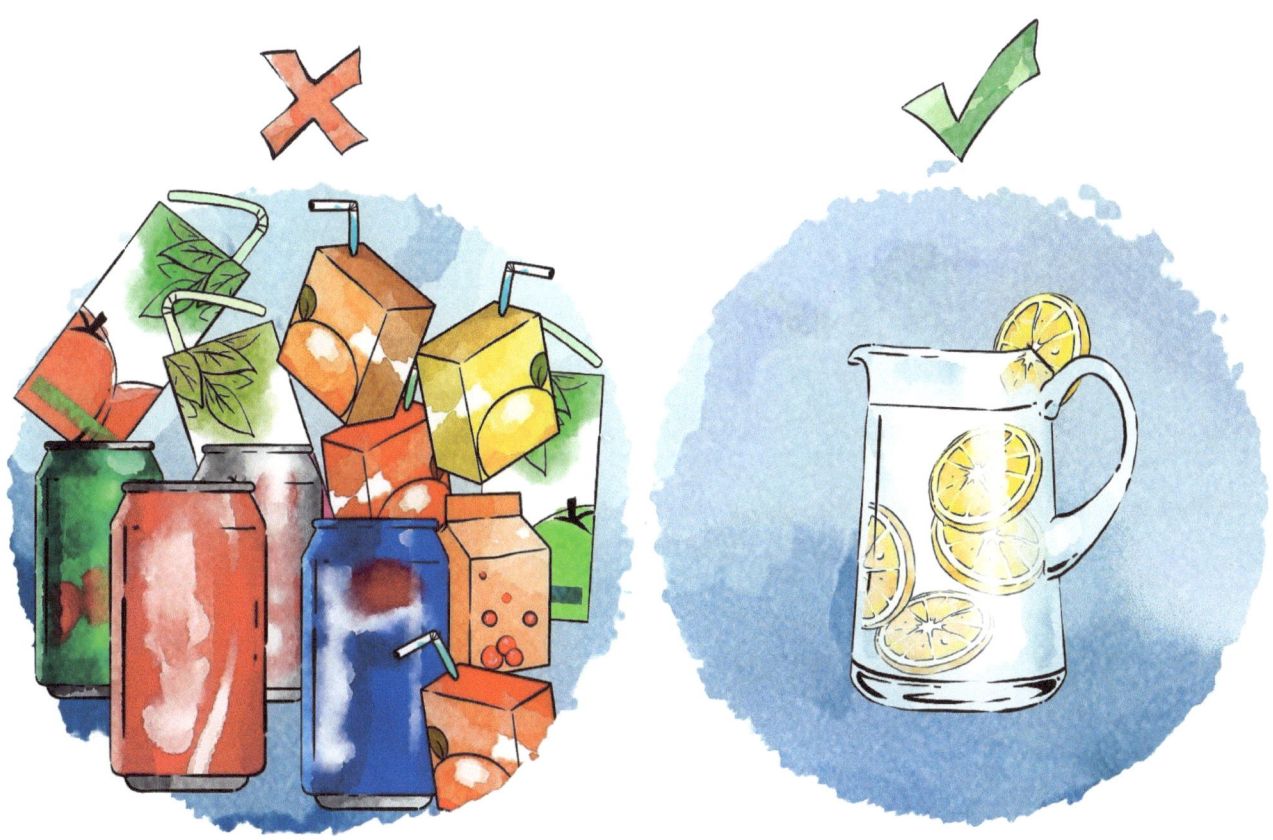

"Water!!" answered the girls with one voice.

"Yes! Pure water keeps you hydrated and is best for your body," Mom confirmed.

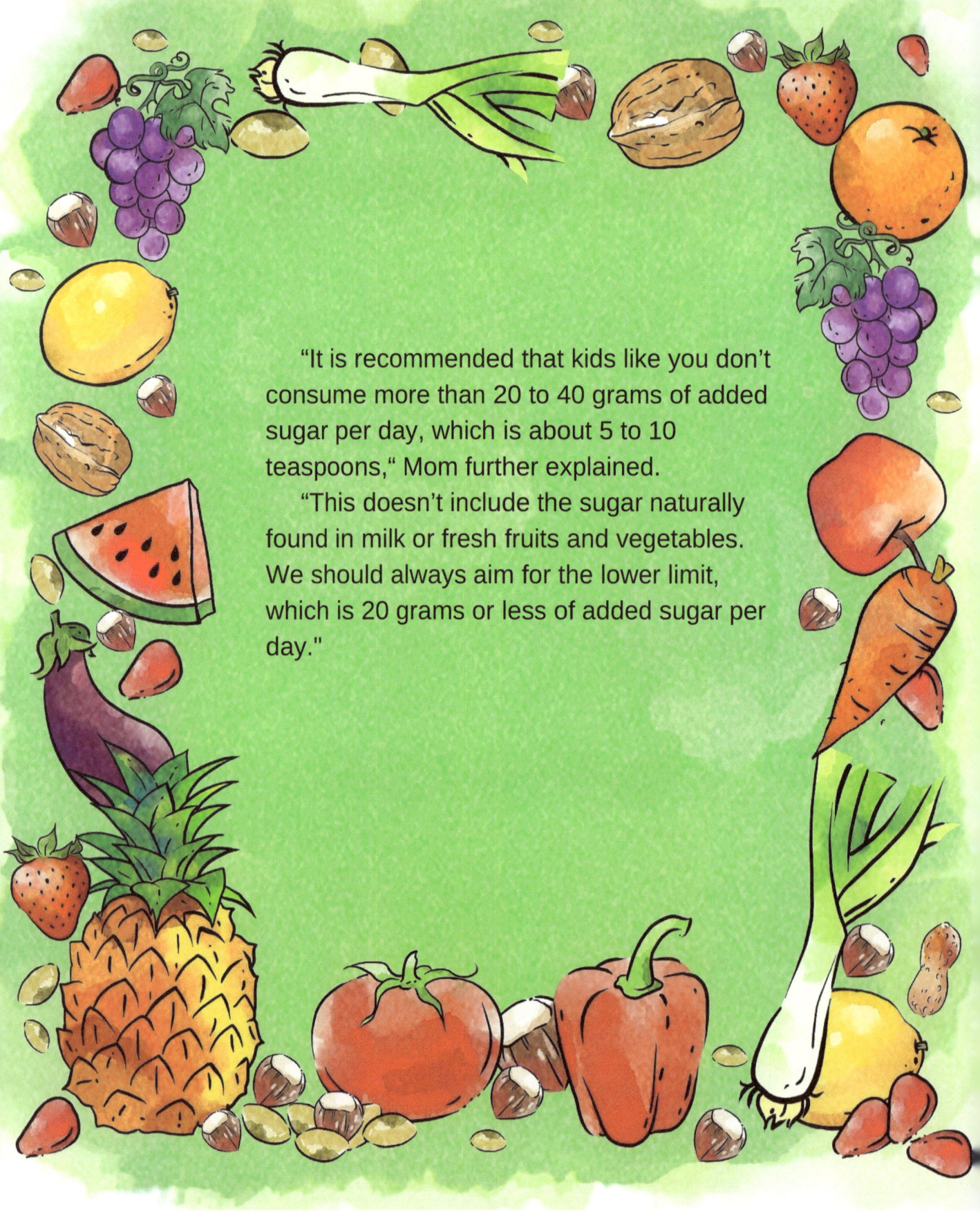

"It is recommended that kids like you don't consume more than 20 to 40 grams of added sugar per day, which is about 5 to 10 teaspoons," Mom further explained.

"This doesn't include the sugar naturally found in milk or fresh fruits and vegetables. We should always aim for the lower limit, which is 20 grams or less of added sugar per day."

"There are many processed foods that we don't think of as sweet, but which contain added sugar, such as ketchup, breads, condiments, sauces, dressings, and crackers. That's why we have to check the labels. These sugars add up quickly and, if we are not careful, we can easily go over the recommended amount," Mom added.

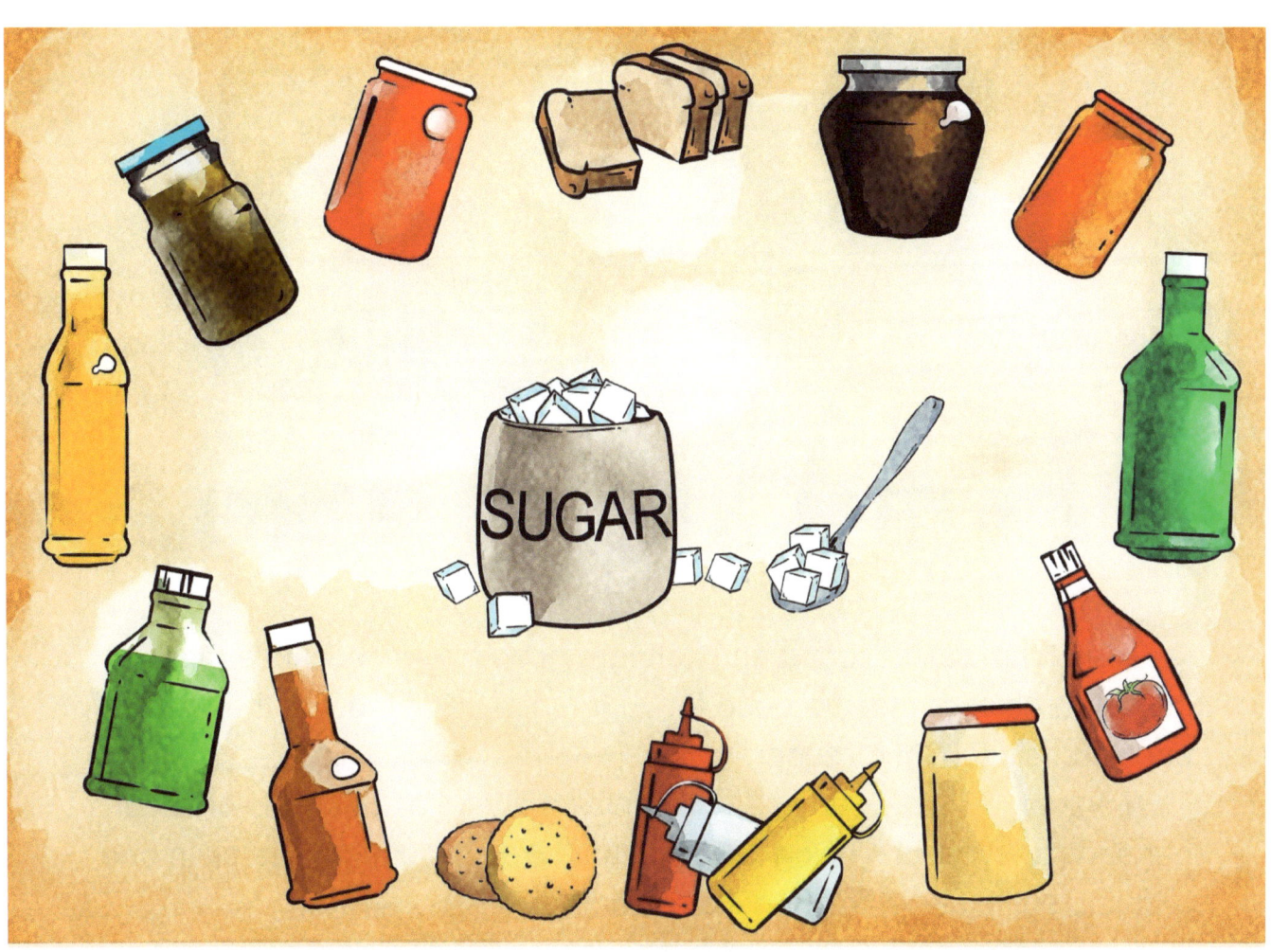

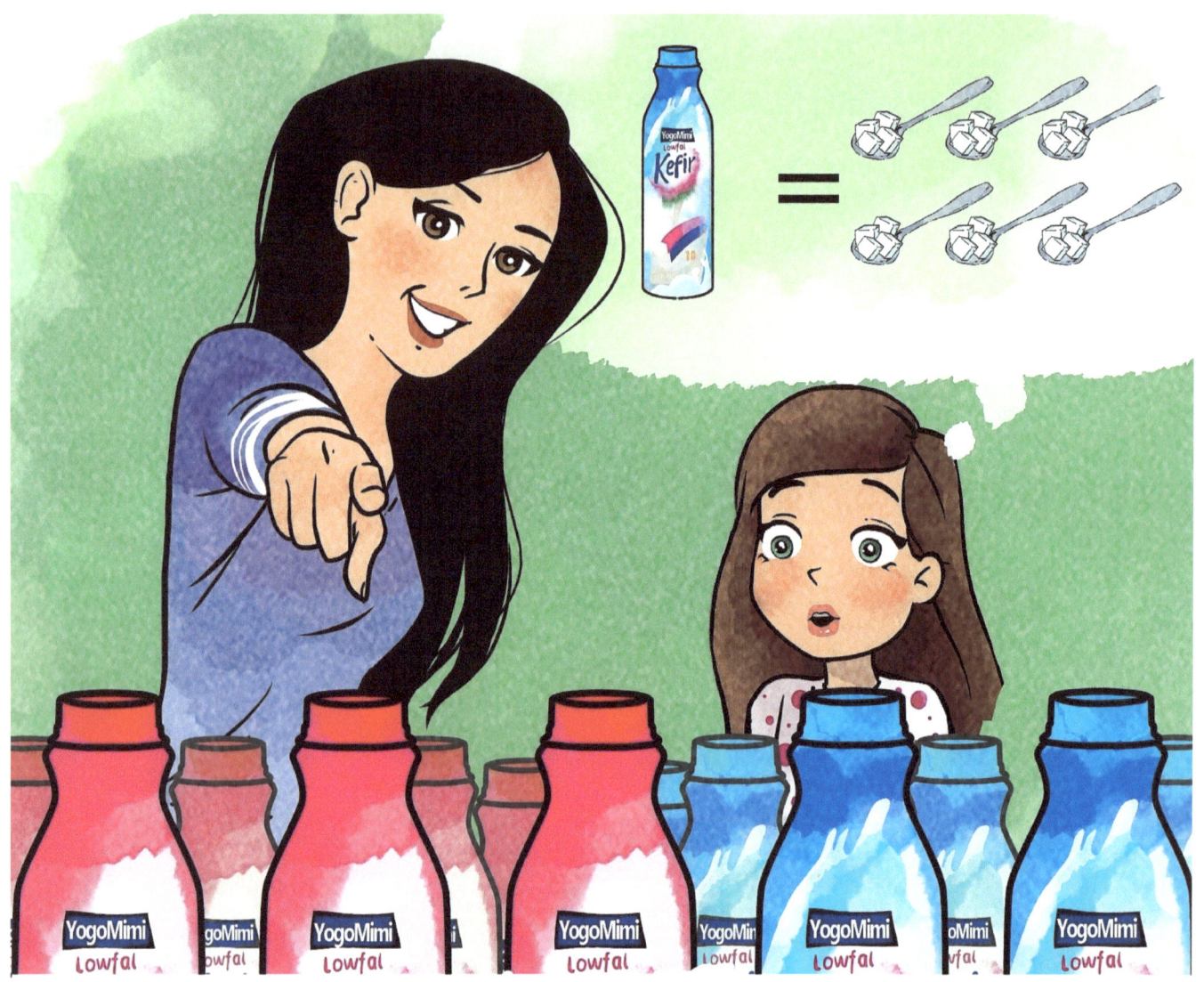

Then Mom said, "Yogurt and kefir are good for you because they contain probiotics that are good for your tummy. But most of the flavored ones contain too much sugar."

"Look at this strawberry kefir: it contains a total of 23 grams of sugar per serving, most of it being added sugar. We can just buy the plain one and add some sweet fresh fruit at home."

"Yes," Maya said, "I love fresh pineapple with goat yogurt!"

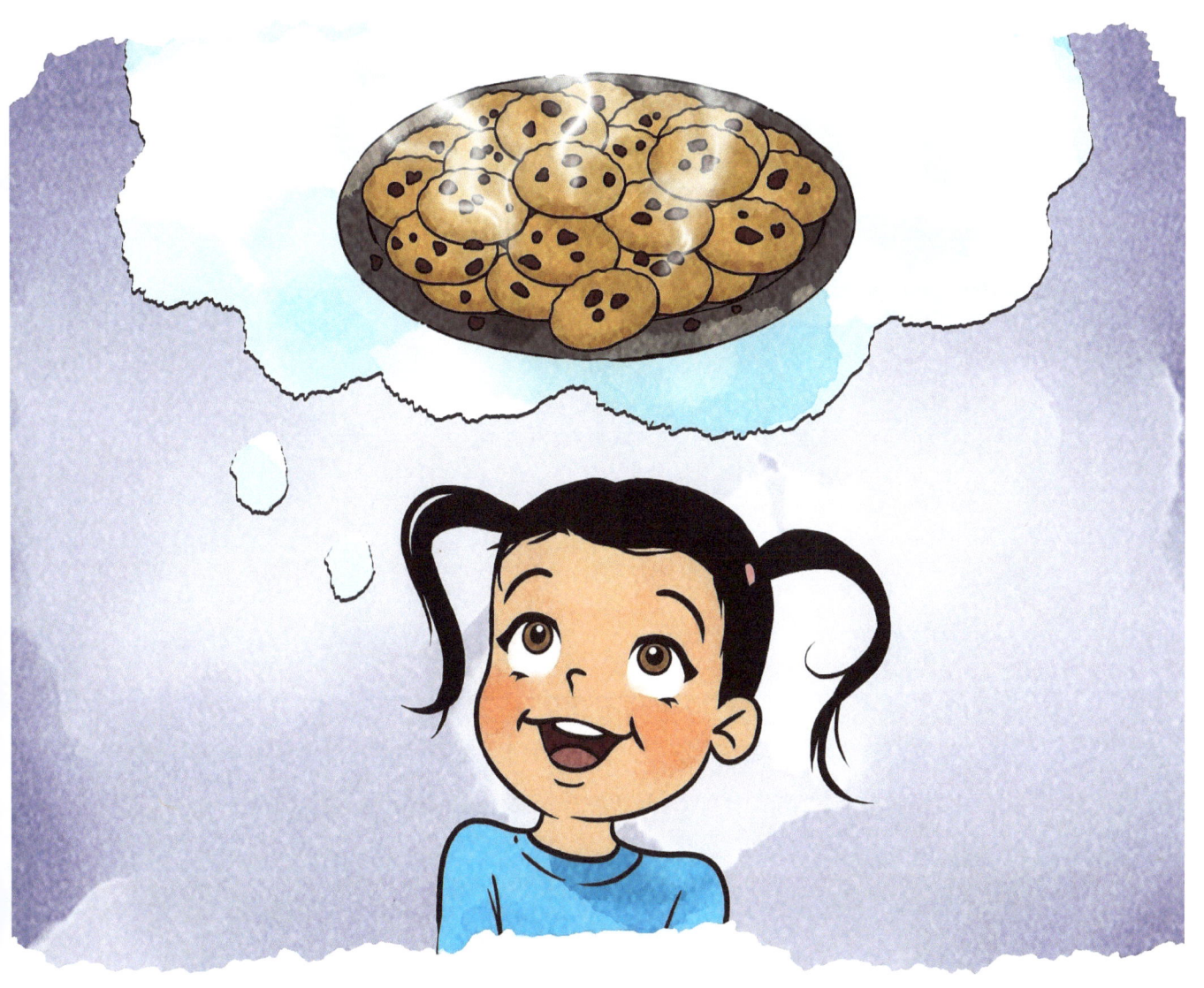

"I prefer that we buy the plain yogurt and no-sugar ketchup and save that sugar to make some yummy cookies this weekend," Zara said.

"I think that's a great idea! We can still enjoy homemade desserts that are made with natural ingredients," Mom agreed.

"We also need to watch out for artificial flavors, sweeteners, and food coloring", Maya said. "Why would we even want to have our food colored?"

"Well," Mom said, "If the food was highly processed, chances are it has a pretty bland look and taste. To sell more of it, food manufacturers add in artificial flavoring, coloring, sweeteners, and too much salt. To avoid these things, it is always a wise choice to stick with real food."

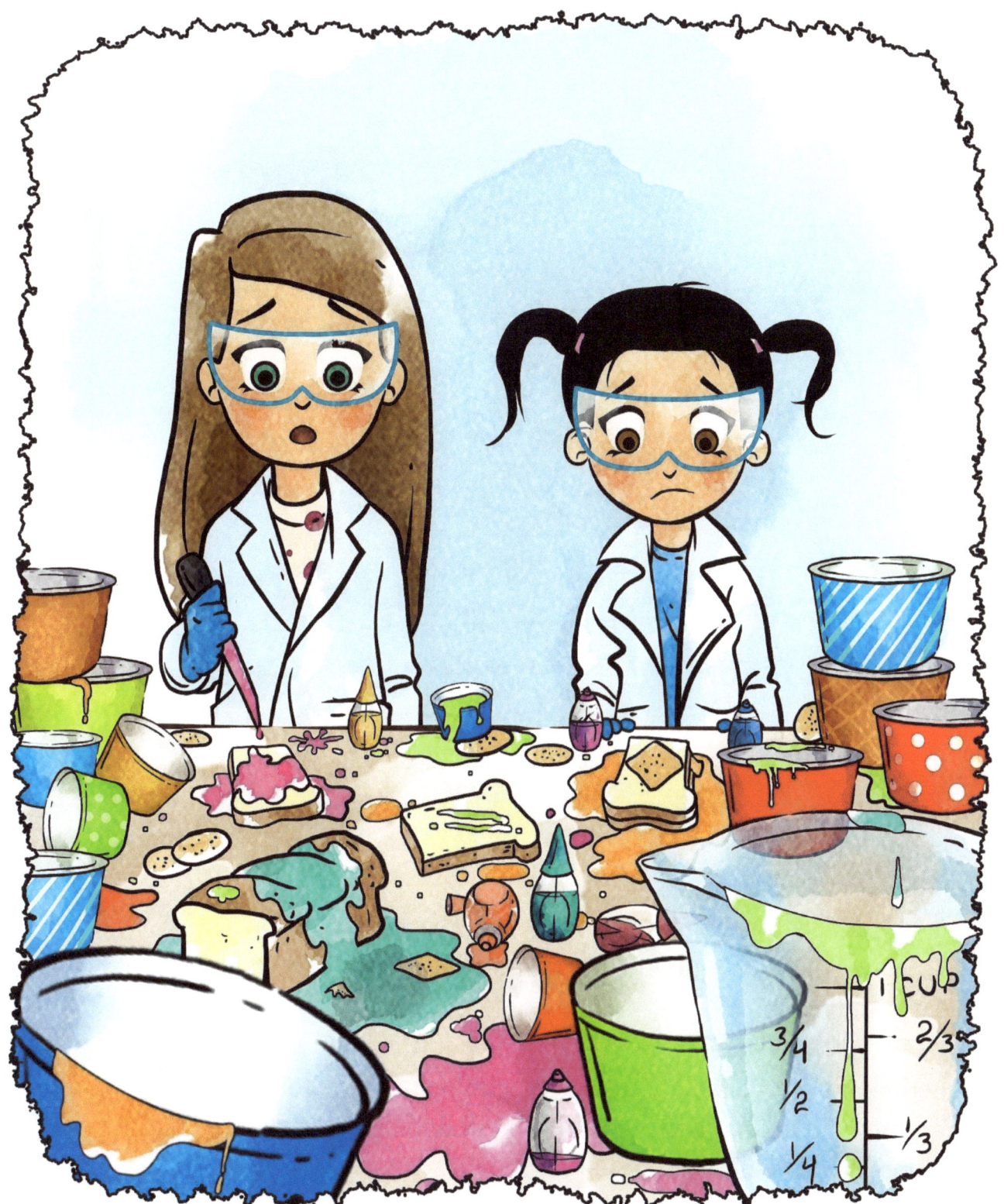

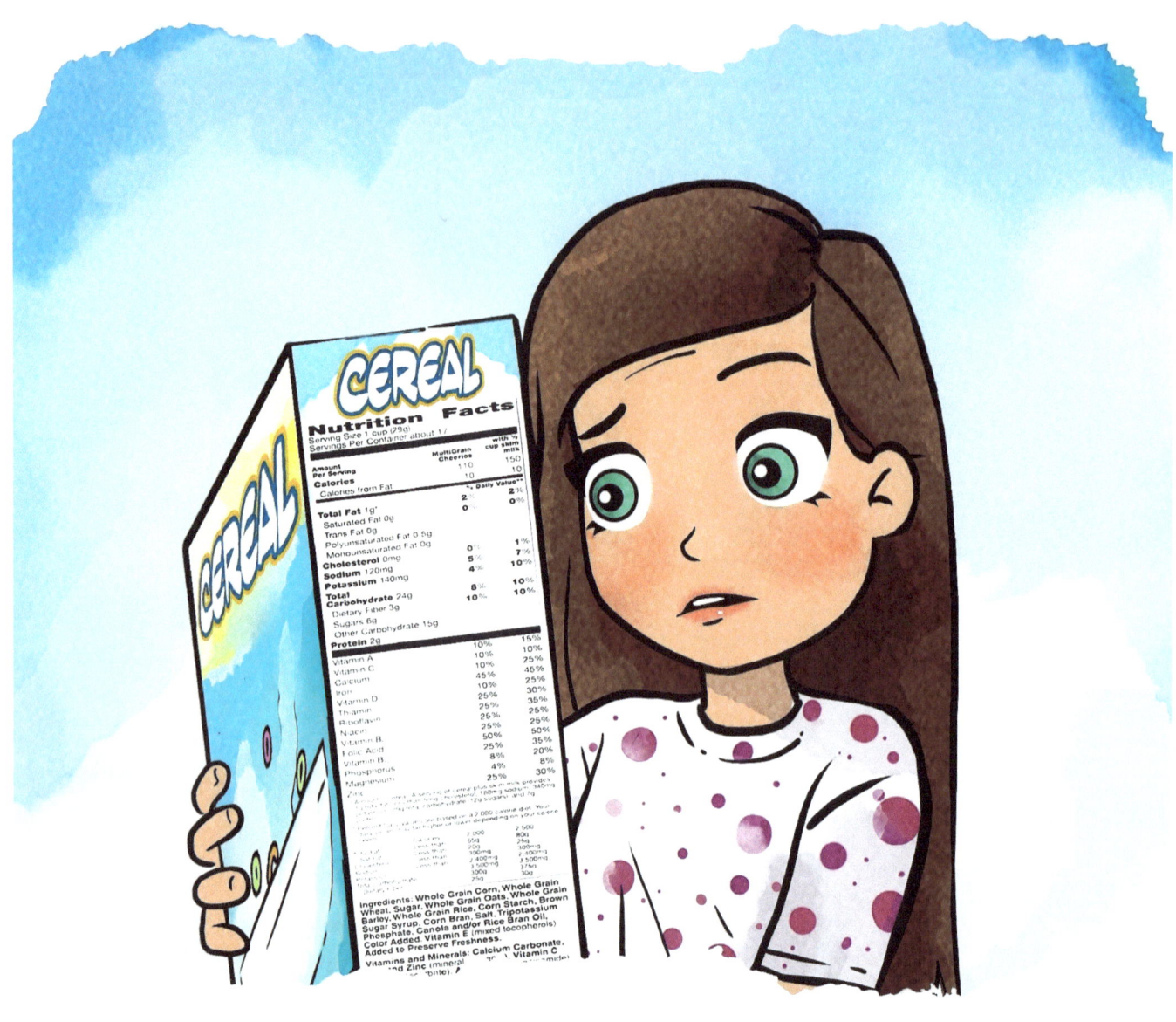

"What else do we need to look for?" Mom asked.

"We want to avoid foods that come with veeery looong ingredient lists," said Maya.

"True," Mom said, "Chances are they contain things you don't want, such as preservatives and additives that would require a chemistry degree to be able to pronounce. What doesn't grow in nature, doesn't belong in your food."

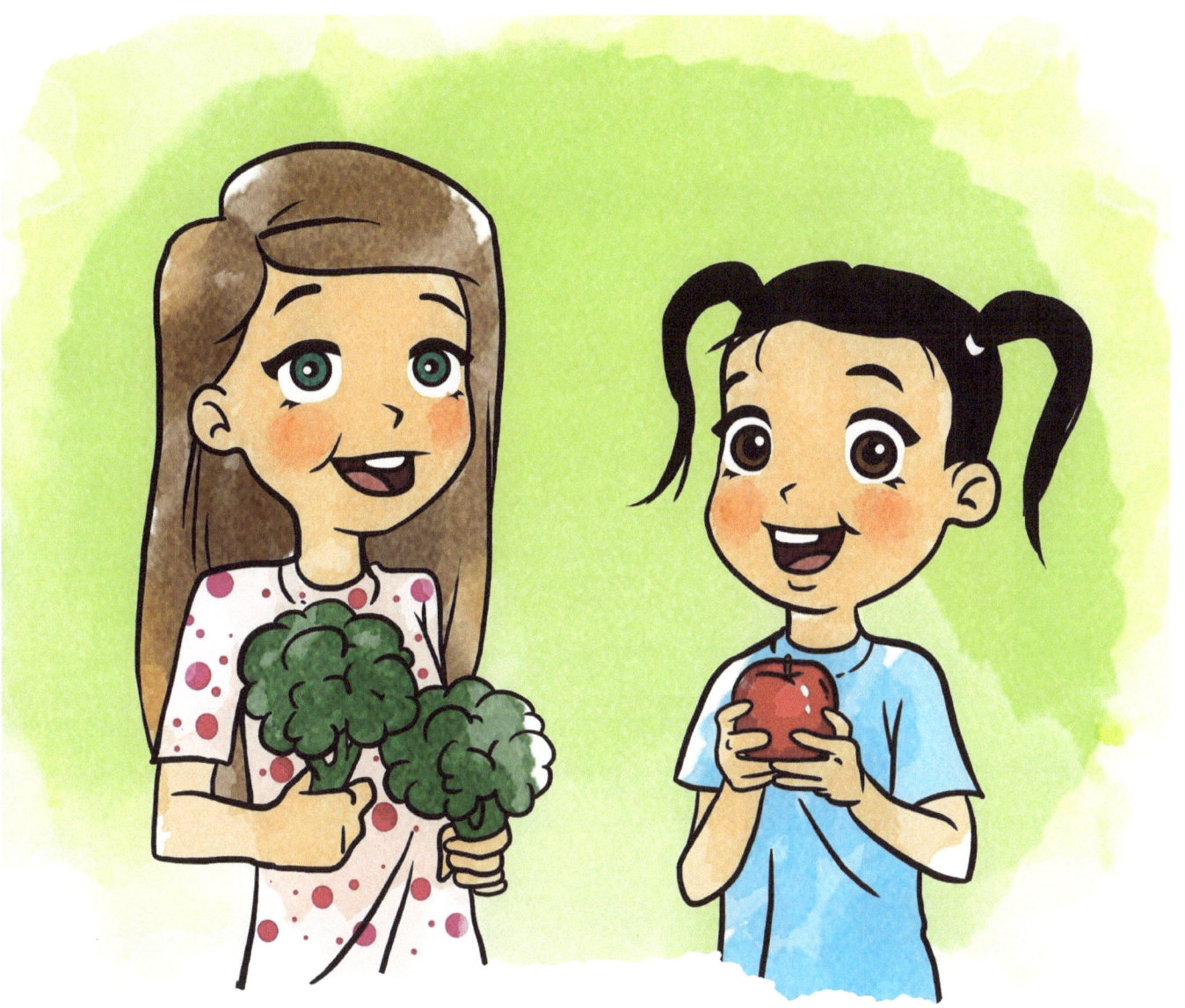

"Does a broccoli bunch need an ingredient list?" Mom asked.

"Noooo..." the girls said, smiling.

"What about an apple?" Mom asked.

"No!" the girls answered again.

"Those are the best foods," Mom said. "Foods that are found in nature don't require an ingredient list and are the best for your body."

"Look, Mom! My favorite pickles!" Maya said.

"And my favorite sauerkraut!" Zara said.

"Those are good because they contain probiotics, which help you to digest foods and make you feel great. But we always check to make sure they contain live or active cultures. This is how we know those probiotics will work for us," Mom says.

"Is this why these jars are in the refrigerated section?" asked Zara.

"Yes," Mom confirmed. "The pickles that are not in the refrigerated section most likely don't contain live cultures."

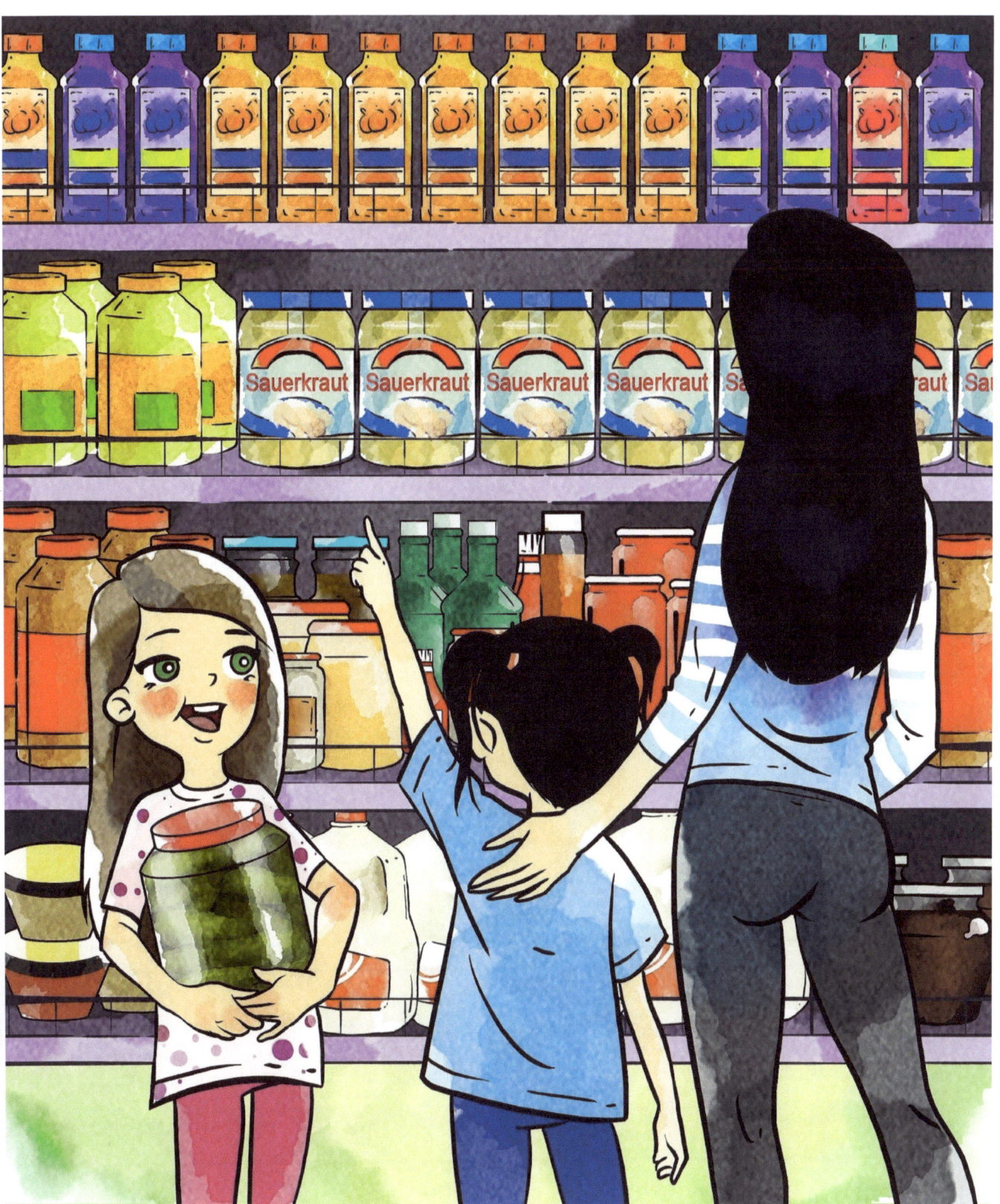

The cart was almost full and it was time to head over to the cash register. The girls were happy to unload the cart and get the bags ready for the food.

"We got everything we needed!" they exclaimed.

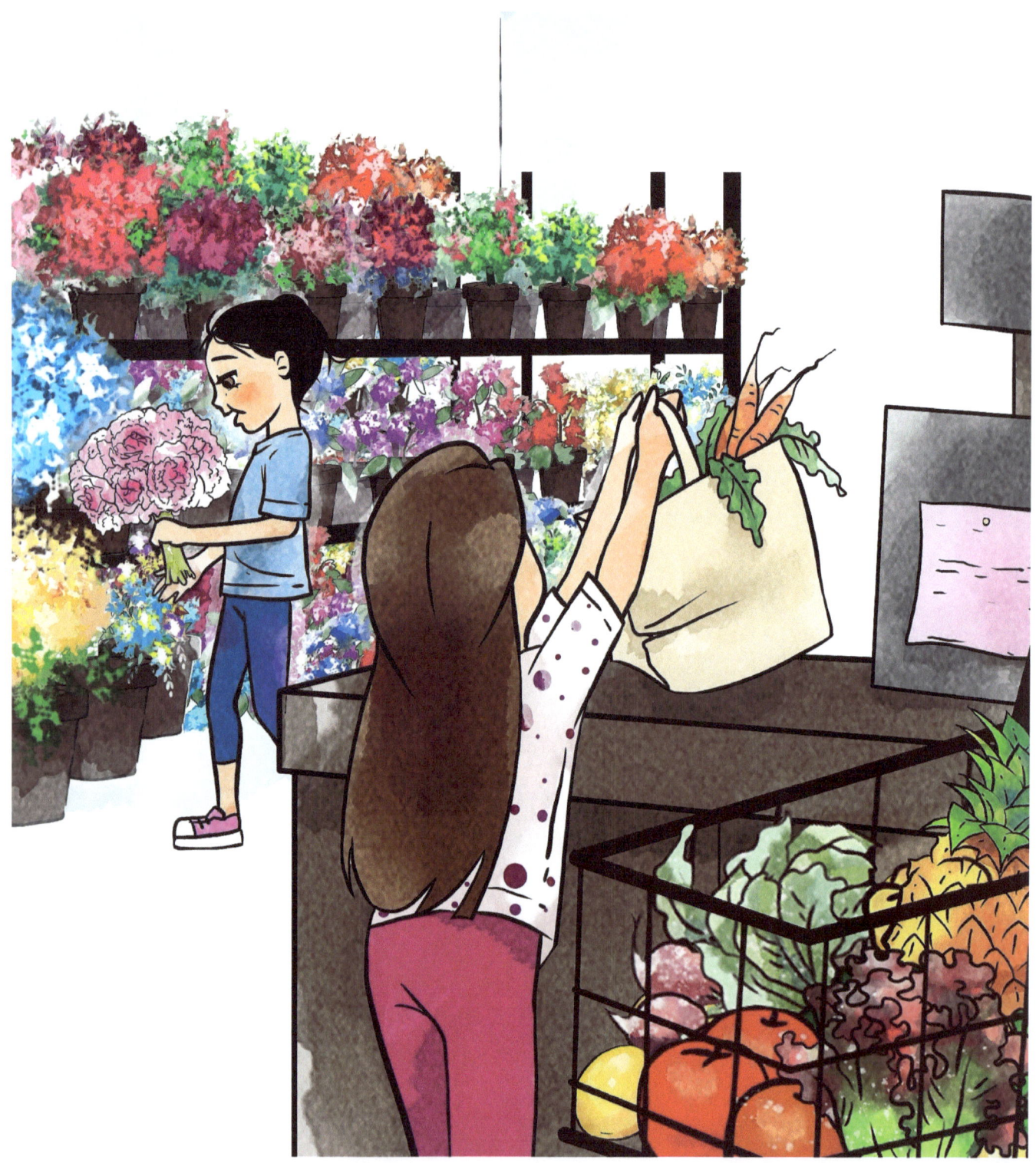

At home, while Mom started to prepare the wild salmon for dinner, the girls were busy baking their favorite cookies.

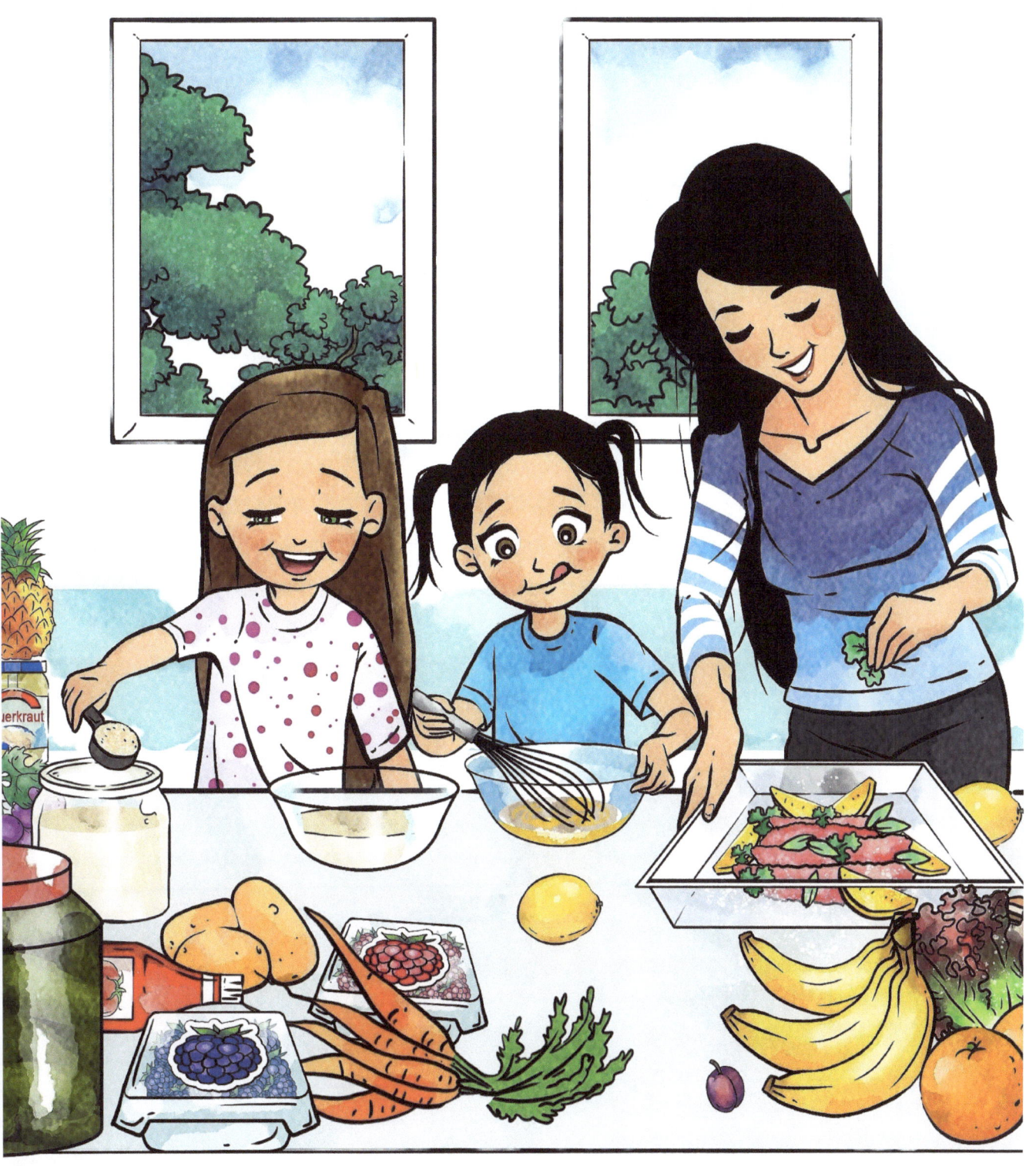

ALMOND CHOCOLATE CHIP COOKIES
~ RECIPE ~

INGREDIENTS:
- 3 cups almond meal/flour
- 1 tsp baking soda
- ¼ tsp sea salt
- 1 tsp vanilla essence
- 5 dried and pitted dates
- ⅓ cup coconut oil or butter, softened
- ¼ cup maple syrup
- 2 eggs
- 1 cup dark chocolate chips

Mix well the almond meal, baking soda, and salt in a bowl and set aside. Put vanilla, coconut oil, maple syrup, dates, and eggs in a blender and blend well until homogenized. Add wet mixture from the blender into the almond meal mixture. Mix well and incorporate the chocolate chips at the end.

Drop the batter by the tablespoon on a baking sheet lined with parchment paper or a silicone baking mat. Bake at 350F (177C) until set and golden, for about 15 minutes.

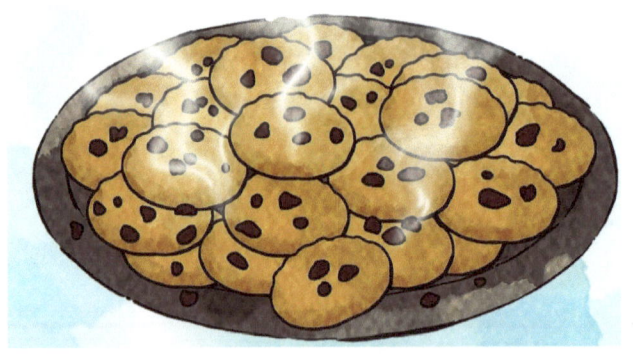

Dinner looked amazing! *Bon appétit!*

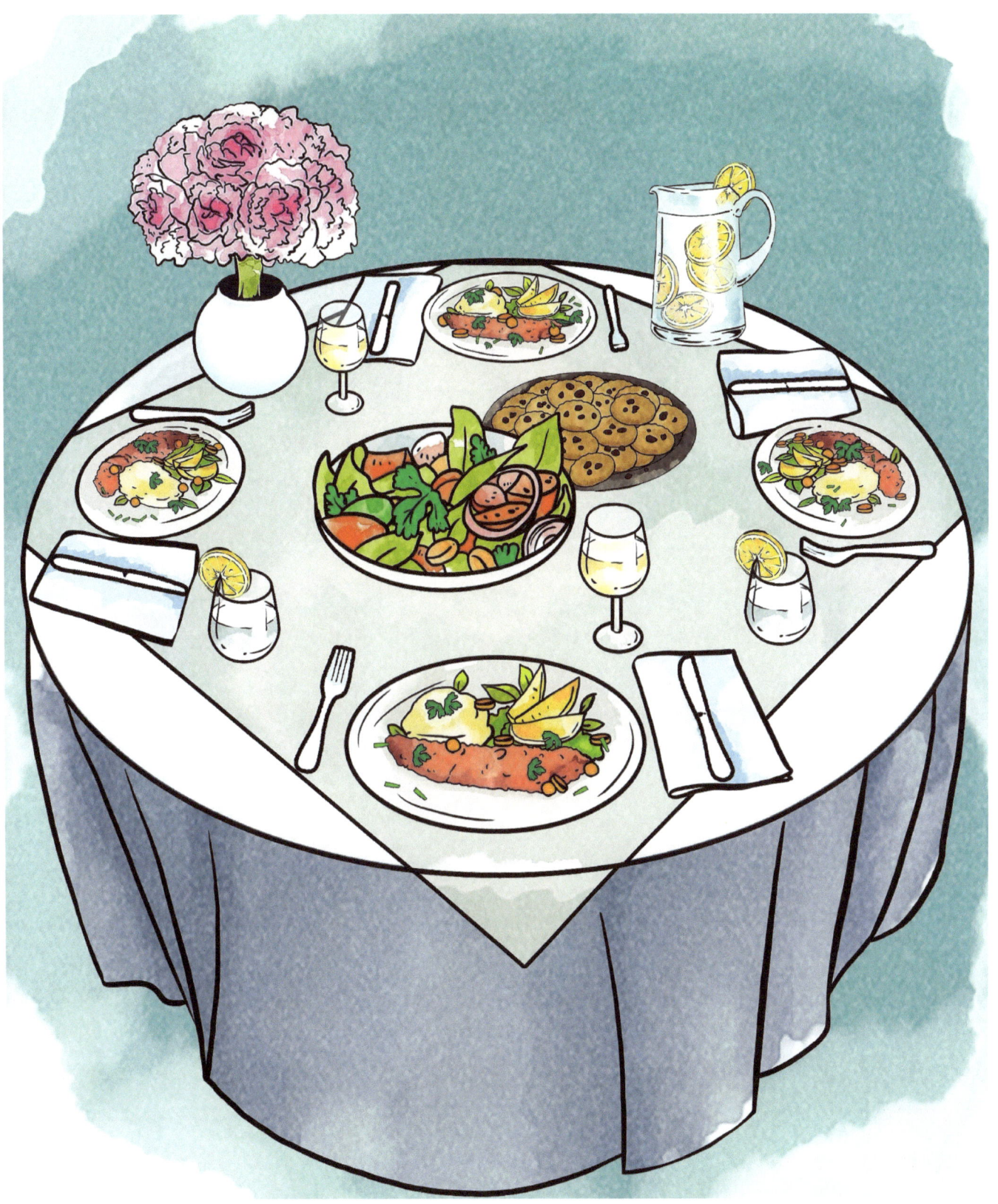

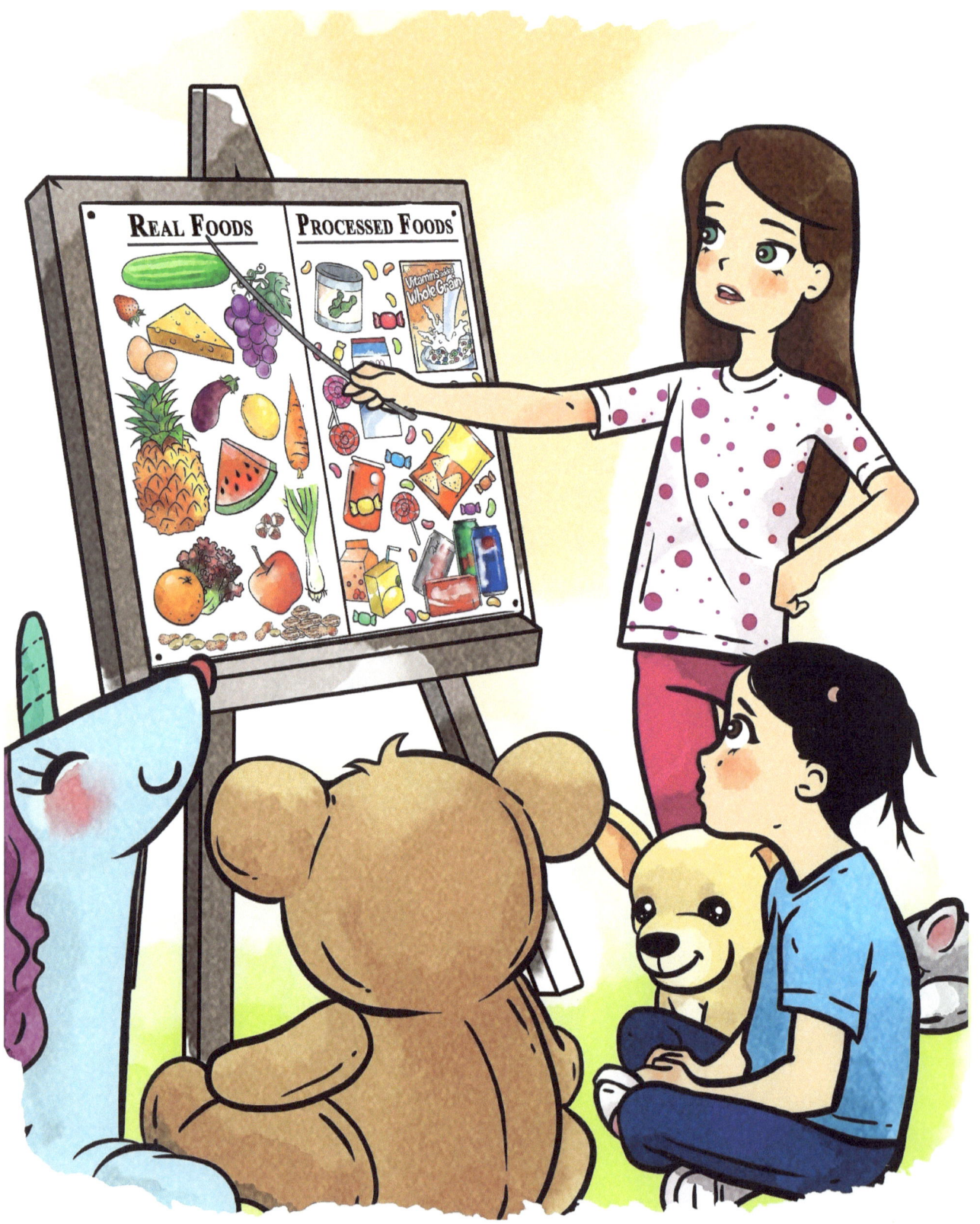

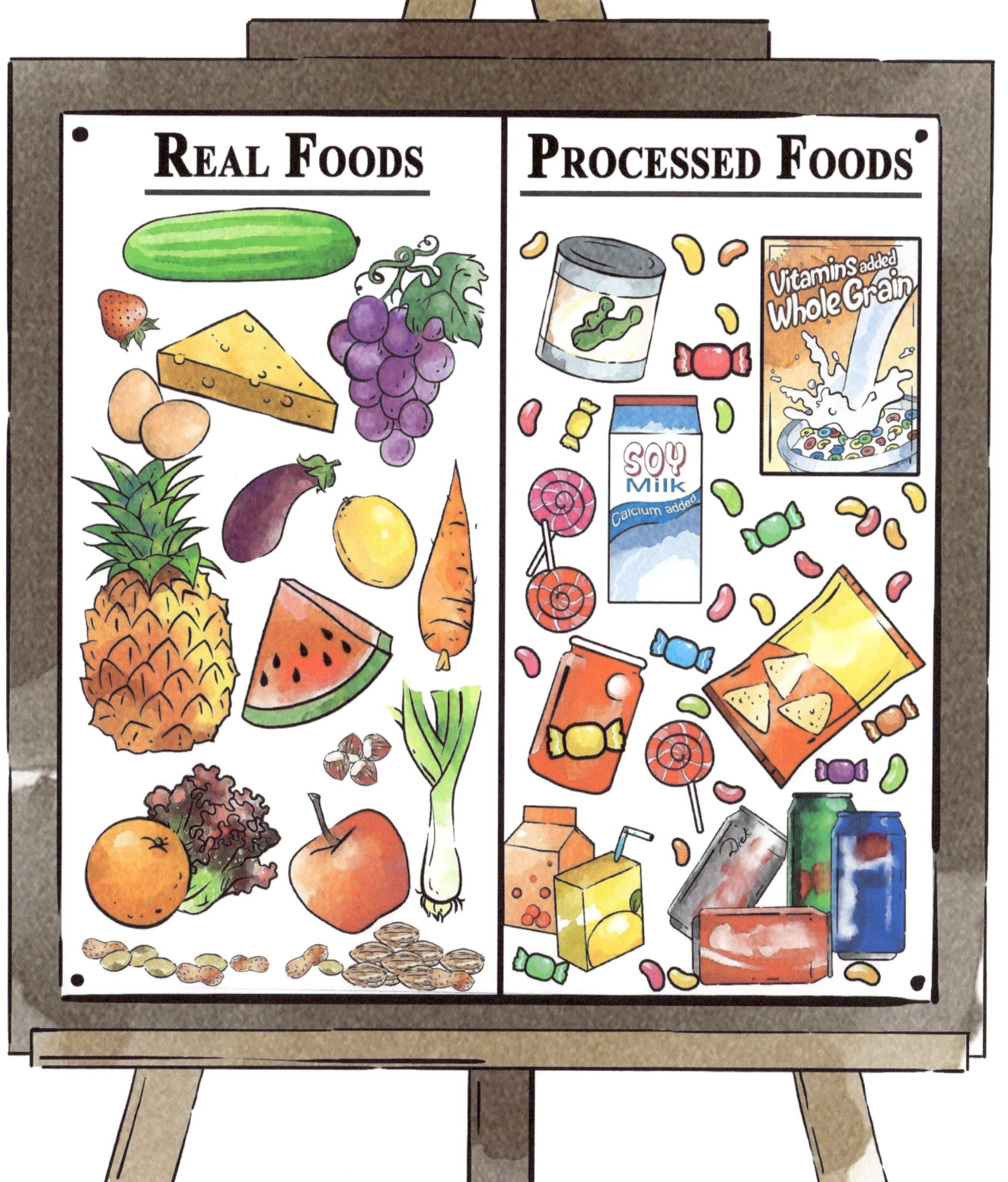

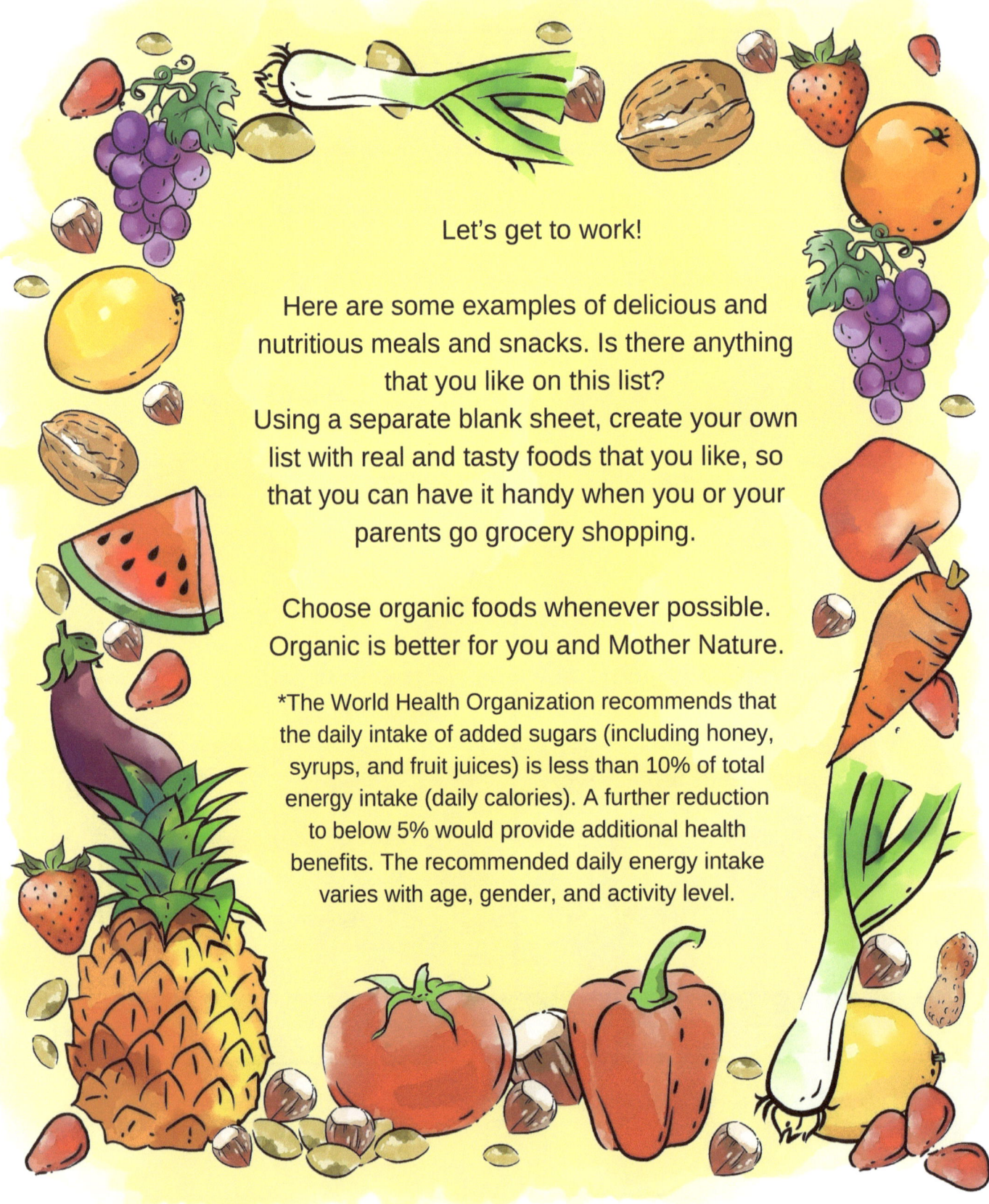

Let's get to work!

Here are some examples of delicious and nutritious meals and snacks. Is there anything that you like on this list?
Using a separate blank sheet, create your own list with real and tasty foods that you like, so that you can have it handy when you or your parents go grocery shopping.

Choose organic foods whenever possible. Organic is better for you and Mother Nature.

*The World Health Organization recommends that the daily intake of added sugars (including honey, syrups, and fruit juices) is less than 10% of total energy intake (daily calories). A further reduction to below 5% would provide additional health benefits. The recommended daily energy intake varies with age, gender, and activity level.

Breakfast

Goat yogurt with berries, pineapple, sliced peaches, or apples and a side of cashews

~ Sunny-side-up eggs with avocado slices and cherry tomatoes

Cooked whole oats with coconut oil, cinnamon, ground walnuts or Brazil nuts, and a touch of raw, unfiltered honey (do not feed honey to babies)

~ Soft or hard boiled eggs, red peppers, and brown rice tortilla

Lunch

~ Whole grain pita bread or spelt tortilla with hummus and cucumbers

~ Lentil & roasted red pepper soup

~ Feta cheese, cherry tomatoes, red onions, olives, and brown rice crackers

~ Chicken noodle soup (try the whole einkorn noodles)

Dinner

~ Roasted chicken with potatoes, rosemary, and green salad

~ Polenta with sour cream, mozzarella cheese, and steamed broccoli

~ Portobello mushrooms, asparagus, quinoa, and garlic sauce

~ Baked wild salmon, steamed and grated cauliflower, and beet salad

Snacks

~ Carrot sticks with hummus

~ Roasted olive oil seaweed

~ Apple slices with almond butter

~ Pickles (with active cultures)

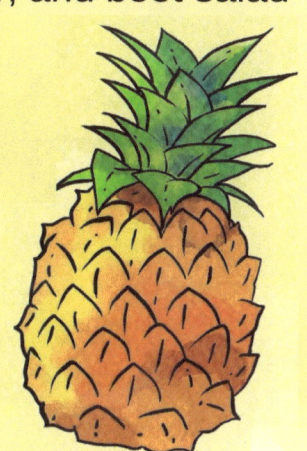

Florentina Marcu is a health coach and mom, living with her family on the outskirts of Los Angeles. Her daughters, Maya and Zara, are her inspiration for this book and her reason for sharing this message of health. For recipes and more health tips, please visit her website at: www.YourHolisticWay.com.

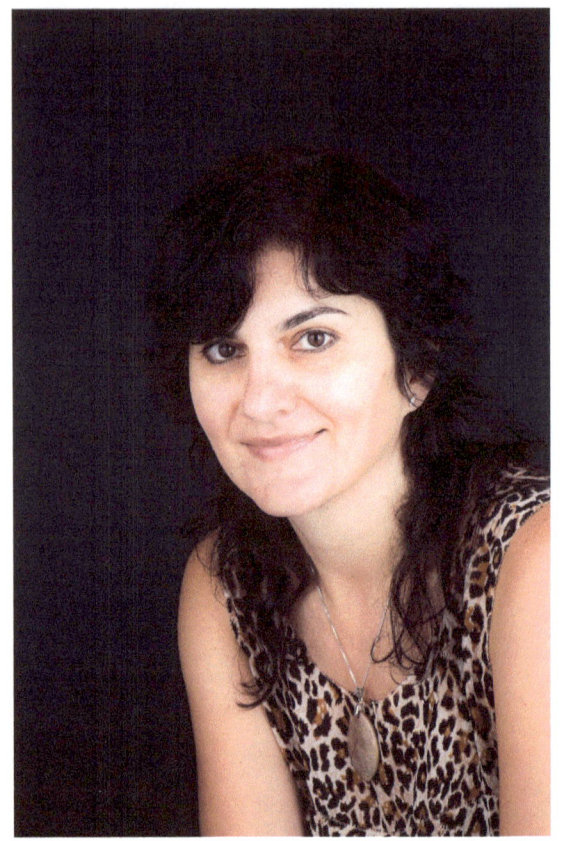

Photo by Sara Jordan

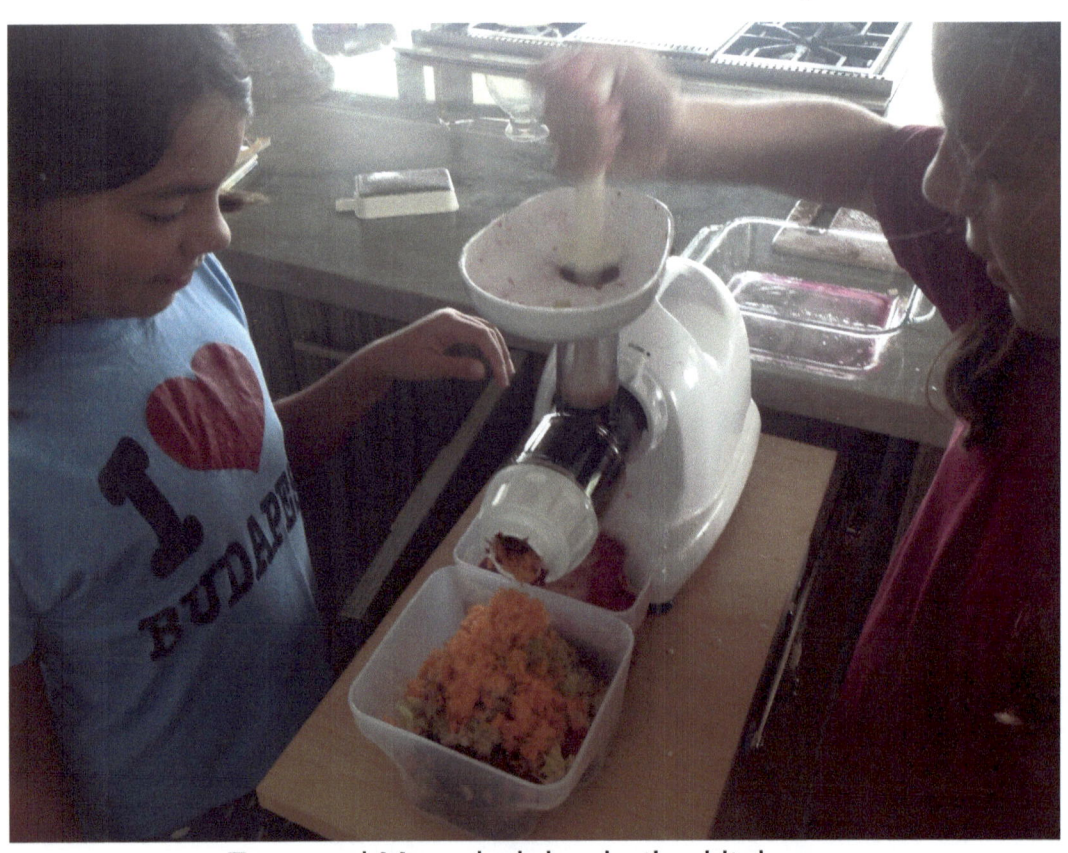

Zara and Maya helping in the kitchen

www.ingramcontent.com/pod-product-compliance
Lightning Source LLC
Chambersburg PA
CBHW041529280526
45792CB00004B/1429